IT's **NOT** A TUMOR!

The Patient's Guide
to
Common Neurological Problems

Robert Wiedemeyer, M.D.

BoxweeD
Publishing

St. Simons Island, Georgia

Although the author and publisher have made every effort to ensure the accuracy and completeness of information contained in this book, we assume no responsibility for errors, inaccuracies, omissions, or any inconsistency herein. Any slights of people, places, or organizations are unintentional. This book is designed to provide information in regard to the subject matter covered. Most of the statistics presented are based on the author's personal experiences and may not coincide with statistics from others in the same profession. Readers should use their own judgment or consult their personal physicians for specific applications to their individual problems.

Wiedemeyer, Robert.
    It's not a tumor!: the patient's guide to common neurological problems / by Robert Wiedemeyer.
        p. cm.
        Includes index.
        Preassigned LCCN: 95-78076.
        ISBN 0-9647407-9-6

1. Neurology—Popular works. 2. Nervous system—Diseases—Popular works. I. Title.

RC346.W54 1996   616.8
                                                  QBI95-20290

ATTENTION ORGANIZATIONS AND INDIVIDUALS: Quantity discounts are available on bulk purchases of this book. Please contact the publisher at the address given above, or call (912) 265-9055, or FAX (912) 261-0085.

PREFACE

After over ten years of treating patients with neuro-logic problems, two things have become glaringly obvious. First, patients seem to be convinced that if their symptoms are related to the nervous system, death is imminent. Second, neurologists have a tendency to perpetuate this myth.

Most diseases of the nervous system are not life threatening. In fact, many neurologic symptoms either require only minimal treatment or no treatment other than reassurance for the patient. When a patient sees a neurologist for headaches, for example, he or she is likely concerned that there is an underlying brain tumor as a cause for the headaches. When the neurologist orders CAT scans, MRIs, and a multitude of blood tests, this reinforces the patient's anxiety. Tumors in the brain can cause headaches; however, I have yet to see a patient with headaches as an only symptom who was later found to have a brain tumor as their cause.

In these times of frequent malpractice litigation, it is more self-protective for physicians to order all of the above tests to verify their findings than to rely solely on the examination of the patient to make a diagnosis.

This book is not intended to be a textbook of diseases related to the nervous system, as most of the information in a neurology textbook applies to less than 1% of the neurologic diseases actually seen in the typical patient with neurologic symptoms. Rather, this book is intended to explain the causes and mechanisms, as well as the treatments, for the most common neurologic symptoms seen by the neurologist in his or her everyday practice. Some of the mechanisms of the functions and malfunctions of the nervous system that are explained in this book are still theoretical, but will almost certainly be proved to be true in the future.

It is hoped that after reading this book, you will be able to recognize the causes for common neurologic symptoms and therefore save yourself some anxiety and possibly even some money.

The Author

CONTENTS

INTRODUCTION
An Overview Of
The Nervous System

The nervous system is composed of two parts, the central nervous system and the peripheral nervous system. The central nervous system consists of the brain and the spinal cord. The peripheral nervous system consists of all the rest of the nerves, including those in the arms, legs, skin, and all other parts of the body, as well as the internal organs, such as the intestines, heart, and lungs.

NERVES

The components of the nervous system are simply living "wires". They conduct actual electric currents from one place to another. Like electric wires, they have central cores which are covered with insulation. There are several million of these wires throughout the nervous system.

Although it may seem elementary, it is worth pointing out that every neurologic symptom or disease is caused by a malfunction in either the insulation or the core of these "wires". For instance, multiple sclerosis, a fairly well known neurologic disease, is caused by defects in the insulation of these "wires".

It has been said that if all the parts of the body were stripped away except for the nerves, you would still be able to recognize all the features of a particular person. Nerves are everywhere. It is this sometimes unfortunate circumstance that is responsible for such diffuse and far reaching symptoms associated with neurologic disease.

A nerve is a bundle of individual "wires", or "neurons". (I will continue to use the term "wire", rather than "neuron", since a wire is much easier to visualize than a neuron.) The wires carry information in one of three directions. They either carry information towards the brain, away from the brain, or from one part of the brain to another part of the brain. When you wiggle your finger, this is information being carried away from the brain towards the muscle that moves the finger. When you cut your finger and feel pain, this pain is information that is carried from your cut finger towards your brain. When you add 23 + 21 mentally, this is information that is being carried from one part of the brain to another part of the brain.

As mentioned above, a nerve is made up of either a few, or several, wires. Some of these wires may be carrying information towards the brain (sensory wires), and some may be carrying information away from the brain (movement wires). If one of these nerves is injured, or cut, then not only would it be possible to lose sensation, but one may also lose the ability to move the part of the body that this particular nerve affects.

One might wonder how the current starts to flow in the first place since there is no "battery" in our bodies. Each wire contains a mechanism by which it can be stimulated. This can be in the form of a heat receptor that, if stimulated, such as by touching a hot stove, will start the current flowing towards the next wire in the sequence. There are also mechanoreceptors that respond to stretching to get the current flowing. Light receptors, such as in the eyes, depend on light for stimulation of the wires in order to get the current flowing towards the brain. These are all examples of peripheral receptors because they are located at the very ends of nerves. All other current in the wires is begun by chemicals that are released from electrically activated wires that stimulate the current to flow from that wire to the next wire in the sequence. These chemicals that cause the current to flow from one wire to another are called neurotransmitters. Different parts of the nervous system use different types of these chemicals. Diseases of the nervous system that affect certain of these chemicals can cause neurologic symptoms. For example, some types of migraine headaches are caused by a lack of a specific chemical in some of the nerves that go to blood vessels around the head. Replacement of this missing chemical can correct the problem and eliminate the headaches.

The current carried over the wires in the body travels much slower than in real electric wires. The largest wires in the body can carry the current at a speed of about 200 miles per hour, and the smallest wires carry the current at about 25 miles per hour. Real electric wires carry current at 669,600,000 miles per hour. Some neurologic diseases cause a slowing in the velocity that current is carried along the wires which can result in a variety of symptoms, depending on which part of the nervous system is involved.

The length of the wires in the central and peripheral nervous systems varies widely, as does the diameter of the various wires.

The shortest wires are only a fraction of an inch in length, while the longest can be 3 to 4 feet in length. The shortest wires usually carry information sideways, such as from one part of the brain or spinal cord to a neighboring part. The longer wires tend to carry information up or down the nervous system, such as between the brain and the spinal cord, or between the spinal cord and one of the extremities.

The diameter of the wires affects the speed at which the wires can transmit information from one point to another. The greater the diameter of the wire, the faster the information travels. The wires with the largest diameters move muscles, such as in the legs and arms. The smallest diameter wires carry information relating to such things as pain and temperature. When you remove your hand from a hot stove and feel most of the pain only after several seconds, this is because it takes the pain information a longer time to reach the brain than the reflex action that makes you remove your hand from the hot surface.

THE BRAIN

The brain generally consists of three main parts. These are the cortex, the subcortex, and the cerebellum.

The cortex is the most advanced part of the brain and is what separates us from the lower animals. It is responsible for thinking, initiating voluntary movement, being aware of all that goes on around us through our five senses, and determines our individual personalities. Diseases that affect the cortex will consequently cause problems in our ability to think, initiate movements, perceive what is going on around us, and may change our personalities. One of the most common causes of malfunction in the cortex is a stroke. A stroke is the result of depriving part of the brain of blood, either because of a blockage in a blood vessel in that part of the brain, or because of a tear in the blood vessel that allows the blood to leak out before it can get to the part of the brain that it normally supplies.

The brain relies on a constant flow of blood to obtain the nutrients and oxygen it needs to live, unlike the rest of the body, which can store nutrients in the form of fat cells and glycogen, a storage form of carbohydrates. On the surface, this may seem like a defect in our "design", since the brain is so important in that it controls everything, and makes us who we are. It would seem that there should be a way to keep the brain supplied with nutrients even when they are not readily available by way of the blood, such as occurs when someone has a stroke.

The answer to this dilemma is probably the lesser of two evils. If the brain were able to store nutrients, these nutrients would have to occupy space in the brain. Unfortunately, the skull is unable to expand and if we filled our skulls up with fat cells and glycogen, there would be no room left for the brain. Also, when parts of the body other than the brain are deprived of oxygen, they are able to obtain energy from nutrients by a different process that, although it is not as efficient as using oxygen, gets the job done. Unfortunately, this process produces by-products, such as lactic acid, that are very toxic to the brain, but don't cause much of a problem in other parts of the body.

The subcortex lies below the cortex. It acts as a kind of "gatekeeper" for the cortex. When information is traveling towards the cortex from the outlying areas of the body, the subcortex filters out unnecessary information and only sends the important information to the cortex for further processing. This keeps the cortex from bogging down. For instance, when you are concentrating on performing some task, such as balancing your checkbook, you are probably less aware of the title of a song that may be playing on the radio in the background than if you were sitting in an easy chair doing nothing with the same song playing in the background.

The subcortex also modifies incoming information so that it is processed easier by the cortex. This may be likened to some of the computer programs that have been developed to make computers more "user friendly".

All information that travels away from the brain is for the purpose of moving muscles. This may pertain to moving individual muscles or large groups of muscles. The subcortex also modifies these outgoing electrical impulses so that when the muscles actually move, they will do so in a smooth fashion rather than in a jerking or flinging way. Diseases that affect the subcortex are usually more notable when they affect this outgoing information from the cortex. For example, Parkinson's disease affects one of the small parts of the subcortex that processes outgoing information from the cortex. Because of the disease process in this small part of the subcortex, patients with this disease have very stiff muscles and tremors of the muscles. Diseases that have abnormal movements as symptoms more often then not are caused by problems in the subcortex. (The subcortex also includes the brainstem.)

Strokes can also occur in the subcortical areas just as in the cortex. If the stroke is in an area of the subcortex that processes incoming information, the patient may have the same type symptoms that he or she would have from a cortical stroke, since the information is being interrupted before it is able to be processed by the cortex. Sometimes after a stroke in the subcortical area, incoming information is jumbled up before it reaches the cortex. This can result in "wrong" information reaching the cortex. For instance, a rare (fortunately) type of subcortical stroke affects the part of the subcortex that processes pain signals. When this type stroke occurs in the subcortex, a patient will feel like he or she is experiencing severe pain in various parts of the body, even though there is nothing wrong with these particular parts of the body. If a subcortical stroke affects outgoing information, the patient may have a weakness on the side of the body affected by those particular wires, or he or she may have an abnormal type movement of the muscles affected by the damaged wires, such as flinging movements, tremors, or writhing type movements.

The third part of the brain, the cerebellum, has been referred to as the modulator of the brain. Its sole purpose has always been thought to be for control of all muscle movement such that our muscle movements will be smooth in motion, both at rapid and slow pace. Without the cerebellum, our movements would look like the type movements a crane used for buildings makes. That is, we would constantly have to keep correcting for overshooting such as when attempting to pick up a pencil. Although the subcortex modifies movements also, as stated above, the cerebellum performs the bulk of this job. It can not perform any of its modulating functions, however, unless the cortex first sends a signal down one of the wires for it to act upon. This is why people with cerebellar diseases have no problems until they try to move.

Without the cerebellum, which sits below the cortex and behind the subcortex, one would be unable to play a piano, strum a guitar, or finger a violin. A surgeon would not be able to perform delicate operations, nor would we be able to drive cars.

Diseases that affect the cerebellum cause problems with smooth movement. For instance, when people have strokes in the cerebellum, they may not be able to feed themselves any longer because of an inability to place food on a fork or spoon and carry it to the mouth without spilling it all before reaching the mouth. It may also be difficult to "find" the mouth as the hand jerks more from side to side as one gets closer to the target. A person's speech may also be affected by a cerebellar problem. Not only may the speech be tremulous with a vibrato characteristic, but it may be explosive as well. That is, the volume of the speech may increase suddenly and then decrease suddenly due to lack of modulation by the cerebellum.

THE SPINAL CORD

After leaving the brain, the next level of importance in the nervous system is the spinal cord. The spinal cord is arranged in small bundles of wires, some of which carry information down the spinal cord to move muscles, some of which carry information up the spinal cord to let the brain know what is going on with the rest of the body, and a third type that doesn't carry information up or down the spinal cord, but rather, sideways.

These wires that carry information sideways let one part of the spinal cord know what another part of it is doing so that the two sides of the body can work synchronously. For instance, while walking barefoot, if someone suddenly steps on a sharp object, he or she will reflexively pick up the foot. At the same time, the opposite leg must tense up to support the entire weight of the body, or the person would fall over. Information traveling sideways in the spinal cord lets the opposite side of the spinal cord know what is going on so it can tell the leg on that side to tense up in order to support the entire body and prevent the person from falling. (The brain itself plays a role in this phenomenon as well, but the spinal cord "assists" in this action.)

Diseases that affect the spinal cord can cause many of the same kinds of symptoms that occur with diseases of the brain, since the spinal cord is the "messenger" that carries information to and from the brain, and if the messenger is impaired, the message doesn't get transported properly. If the brain only gets part of a message, it can't make an "informed" decision about how to react to this information. For instance, if a person is wounded by a bullet that happens to hit one of the bundles of wires in the spinal cord that carries temperature information from the foot to the brain, the brain will no longer tell the foot to move if it steps on a hot surface because it is no longer aware that the surface is hot.

Although strokes can occur in the spinal cord, the most common cause of malfunction in the spinal cord is traumatic injury, such as from gunshot wounds, diving into pools that are too shallow, and automobile accidents.

PERIPHERAL NERVES

The next level of the nervous system is the peripheral nerves. These make up the bulk of the nervous system and, as stated above, are everywhere in the body except in the brain itself and in the spinal cord itself.

The wires that make up the peripheral nervous system are a little bit different than the ones that make up the brain and spinal cord. For one thing, the insulation on these nerves is slightly different, a feature that makes them susceptible to certain diseases that don't affect the brain and spinal cord, and makes the brain and spinal cord susceptible to diseases that don't affect the peripheral nerves. An example is multiple sclerosis, again, which is a disease that affects the insulation on the wires in the brain and spinal cord, but not the insulation on the wires in the peripheral nerves. A second, and major, difference between the peripheral and central nervous system is that the peripheral nerves are capable of regeneration, to a degree, when they are damaged. If a nerve is damaged in the brain or spinal cord, it is damaged forever. In some cases, when a person has a larger peripheral nerve severed, a surgeon can actually sew the nerve back together and function is eventually restored. Researchers have been trying for years to find a way to get the central nervous system to regenerate when damaged, but so far, have been unsuccessful.

Hopefully, this overview of the nervous system will make it easier to understand some of the mechanisms involved in the various symptoms discussed in the following chapters. If one remembers that every disease affecting the nervous system has its effect on either the core or the insulation of the wires that make up the nervous system, and that the various diseases affect either the brain, the spinal cord, the peripheral nerves, or combinations of these parts, it will be much easier to see how and why various malfunctions in the nervous system can produce the symptoms that we see.

Chapter 1
HEADACHES

The most common cause for visits to a physician is a patient's complaint of headaches. Over 90% of people have headaches and a large number of these people have severe enough symptoms that they are not able to treat them with over-the-counter pain relievers. Some people become plagued by headaches that seem to be present constantly, while others have headaches infrequently but, when they do get a headache, it is incapacitating to the point that the patient has to lie down in a dark room for up to several hours until the pain resolves, or at least becomes more tolerable.

Headaches are caused by one thing and one thing only: irritation of wires around the head that carry pain information to the brain. This irritation can be in the form of compression of these pain carrying wires from muscle spasms or swelling of surrounding tissues, stretching of blood vessels that are surrounded by pain carrying wires, or from abnormal impulses being generated within the pain carrying wire itself.

In my experience, more than 95% of all headaches are

caused by either compression of pain carrying wires from muscle spasms around the head and neck, or from stretching of the pain carrying wires that encircle blood vessels around the head when these blood vessels dilate for one reason or another. The other 5% of headaches would be made up of those that result from compression of pain carrying wires by swelling of surrounding tissue and those headaches that result from abnormal impulses being generated within the pain carrying wire itself.

MUSCLE CONTRACTION HEADACHES

The most common cause of headaches is compression of pain carrying wires from muscle spasms in the area of the head and neck. Again using my experience, about 80% of headaches are from this cause. These are commonly called "muscle contraction headaches". They can occur at various times of the day and can last for as short a period of time as one hour or may be unrelenting over a period of several weeks or months. When a person has a muscle contraction headache, he or she can usually function fairly normally but is more than likely a little irritable. If this type of headache lasts for longer than a week or two, the person will gradually start showing signs of depression. That is, he or she may develop a loss of appetite, begin having difficulty with concentration, and may have trouble falling asleep at night.

Almost everyone has had a muscle contraction headache at one time or another. The most common cause for this type of headache is stress. When a person is under stress, there is increased extraneous electrical activity in the wires of the brain and some of this extraneous electrical activity filters down through the brainstem to the upper spinal cord and then out from the spinal cord to the peripheral nerves that go to the muscles around the head and neck where it causes the muscles to contract. (Remember, all information that leaves the brain is for the purpose of moving muscles, even when it is extraneous information.) In underdeveloped countries where stress, as we know it, is not as high as in more developed countries, muscle contraction headaches are not as common.

There are, of course, other causes of muscle contraction headaches. Loud noises, especially for extended periods of time, can cause this type of headache. The mechanism is much the same as in muscle contraction headaches caused by tension. The constant noise stimulates the receptors in the ears for hearing. This information is then carried over the wires to the brain. The more noise there is, the more information there is for the brain to handle. The excess that is not able to be handled by the brain filters down through the brain to the spinal cord and then out the peripheral nerves to the muscles around the head and neck where it causes them to contract, compressing the pain carrying nerves, thus causing the muscle contraction headache.

Visual problems can also cause muscle contraction headaches. When a person strains, either knowingly or unknowingly, to bring an object into focus over an extended period of time, the muscles around the eyes that are used for this straining ultimately also compress the pain carrying wires which, once the information reaches the brain, is perceived as a headache.

Chronic neck pain can also cause chronic muscle contraction headaches. This is simply because chronic neck pain is usually caused by chronic muscle spasms of the neck. These muscle spasms compress the pain carrying wires and cause headaches in the same way as explained above.

Post concussive syndrome results from a sudden acceleration-deceleration type injury, also called whiplash. People can develop muscle contraction headaches after this type injury from two different causes. The first type results from the neck spasms that occur after a whiplash injury. (The cause of these neck spasms will be explained further in the chapter on neck and back pain.) The second cause for muscle contraction headaches after a whiplash injury relates to a kind of "mixing up" of the chemicals in the brain that control the carrying of information from one wire in the brain to another. This can result in unnecessary (extraneous) electrical information being produced which, as stated earlier, finds its way through the brain, spinal cord, and out the peripheral wires to the muscles of the neck and head, compressing the pain carrying wires, which the brain then perceives as a dull, aching, continuous headache.

In general, a muscle contraction headache is a constant, dull, band-like pain that does not pulsate unless it becomes more severe. It is usually not associated with nausea or vomiting unless, again, it becomes severe.

VASCULAR HEADACHES

The second most common type of headache is the type that results from stimulation of the pain carrying wires that surround blood vessels. These are called "vascular" headaches. In my experience, about 15% of headaches are of this type. The blood vessels that are involved in vascular headaches are the arteries, which carry blood away from the heart to all the parts of the body, (including the head) and which are under very high pressures, as opposed to the veins, which carry blood towards the heart from the various parts of the body, and are under very low pressures. When the pain carrying wires that encircle these arteries become stretched, they send pain information to the brain which the brain perceives as a headache. This stretching, or "dilation", of the blood vessels occurs because of various reasons, including high blood pressure, spasms of the muscular walls of these blood vessels, or from swelling due to inflammation of these blood vessels.

The pain that results from vascular headaches is quite severe. Patients usually complain of a pulsating type pain that coincides with their heartbeats, associated nausea, frequent vomiting, pain in the eyes when in the presence of bright lights, and a need to lie down in a dark room where they may finally fall asleep. Frequently, when the person awakens, the headache is gone but he or she feels very drained and tired for up to several hours afterward. Fortunately, vascular headaches are usually much less frequent in occurrence than muscle contraction headaches. Typically, they will occur every couple months. They may last for a few minutes or up to several hours, but when they finally resolve, there is no lingering pain for several days, except in a few cases, which will be mentioned below.

It is unknown why blood vessels spasm, triggering vascular headaches. One supposed cause, which is most likely accurate, is that small molecules, such as pollen particles, are breathed in through the lungs, find their way into the bloodstream, and then as they get carried around the bloodstream, they trigger blood vessel spasms as they bump into the blood vessel walls. Most people with vascular headaches seem to have more of them during the high pollen seasons, such as in the spring and the fall, which would fit with the above theory as a possible cause for these types of headaches.

True "migraine" headaches are vascular headaches. Most people who complain of chronic "migraine" headaches actually are suffering from a more severe form of muscle contraction headache rather than from a true "migraine". This can be determined by the history of the headaches. If a patient tells me that he or she has had a continuous, severe headache for the last three months, this would fit more with a severe muscle contraction headache than a true migraine headache. (There are some types of vascular headaches that can occur several times a day for a

few weeks. These are called cluster headaches and are relatively rare. They are usually located on one side of the
head and have associated stuffy nose on that same side,
tearing from the eye on that side, and are not continuous.
They may last for 1 or 2 hours, then resolve, only to return
again later that day. This can go on for a few weeks, then
spontaneously resolve until the next attack several months
later.)

There are several types of vascular, or migraine,
headaches. (Vascular and migraine are terms that are often
used interchangeably.) These types include classical
migraine, common migraine, complicated migraine, and
atypical migraine.

Classical migraine is the most well described type of
vascular headache. It begins with some type of visual problem, followed soon thereafter by a severe, pulsating type
headache, usually located over one of the temples. The
visual change usually consists of jagged, bright lights in the
peripheral vision, may consist of squiggly lines in the central vision, blurred vision, or even partial to complete loss
of vision temporarily. These visual symptoms always clear
up after a brief period of time and are followed by the
intense headache. The cause of this sequence of events is
the spasming of the artery on the side of the head that is
involved. First, the artery spasms into the closed position,
which decreases the flow of blood to the eye on that side.
When the eye doesn't get enough blood, it then doesn't get
enough nutrients to function properly, which causes the
visual changes described above. After the artery finishes
spasming in the closed position, after several minutes, it
then begins to dilate. If it would dilate back to its normal
position, there would be no associated headache following
the visual changes. Unfortunately, it dilates well beyond
the normal position, stretching the pain carrying wires that
encircle the artery. These wires send the pain information
to the brain where it is perceived as a headache. After sev-

eral minutes to hours, the artery gradually returns to its normal caliber and the headache resolves.

Common migraine gets its name because it is the most "common" type of migraine. (Classic migraine, although well described in texts over the years, is not really very common.) Common migraine consists of the headache portion of the symptom complex, but without the visual changes. The reason for this is that the artery doesn't spasm closed first, it simply dilates, stretching the pain carrying wires, then returns back to its normal caliber after a period of time. In my experience, about 75% of vascular headaches are common migraines.

Complicated migraine is similar to classic migraine but rather than the spasming of the artery in the closed position causing visual symptoms, the spasms in the closed position are so much stronger that they actually deprive the brain itself from receiving an adequate supply of blood on the affected side. This results in a noticeable numbness or weakness on the opposite side of the body, much like the numbness and weakness associated with strokes. (Each half of the brain controls the opposite half of the body.) Like classic migraine, this spasming closed of the artery is followed by excessive dilation of the artery, resulting in stretching of the pain carrying wires around the artery and hence, the vascular headache. This headache that follows the symptoms of numbness or weakness on the opposite side of the body from the side of the headache is very important to a neurologist taking the patient's history of the events after they have cleared up because it may be the only thing that lets him or her know that this was a complicated migraine rather than a stroke. (A stroke is usually not associated with an accompanying headache.) It may be worth mentioning at this point that some women who are on birth control pills and have a history of complicated migraines are at an increased risk for having actual strokes because some of the birth control pills have a tendency to make the blood a little thicker which, when coupled with the intense spasming of the artery in the closed position during the onset of the complicated migraine, can actually cause a blood clot to form in the constricted area of the artery, preventing any blood from passing beyond that point. When the blood flow stops completely, this is a stroke.

Atypical migraine consists of the spasming of arteries on one side of the head in the closed position, resulting in visual changes, such as in classic migraine, or numbness or weakness on the opposite side of the body, such as in complicated migraine. However, this spasming in the closed position is not followed by excessive dilation of the artery; it simply returns to normal caliber eventually. Atypical migraine is therefore not associated with a headache at all. This type "headache" is very difficult to distinguish from a stroke, (or transient ischemic attack, which is a stroke that completely resolves) because like a usual stroke, there is no associated headache to tip off the neurologist that something else is causing the symptoms. Oftentimes, when a patient has numbness or weakness on one side of the body that resolves over a short period of time, especially in a young person who would not ordinarily be at risk for a stroke, an atypical migraine may be blamed.

Other causes for vascular headaches that don't involve spasms of blood vessels do involve inflammation of the blood vessels around the head. Inflammation is a process that involves several steps, but the only one that is important for purposes of this discussion is "swelling". It is this swelling of the blood vessels when they become inflamed that affects the pain carrying wires that surround the blood vessels. The swelling can affect the pain carrying wires in two ways. First, when the blood vessel swells up, it can mechanically stretch the pain carrying wires, thus causing these wires to send pain information to the brain which the brain perceives as headache. Second, when the individual cells that make up the blood vessel swell from the inflammation process, the walls of these cells are not able to hold all the liquid contained within the cells. Some of it leaks out of the cell and comes into contact with the pain carrying wires. When it touches these wires, it triggers an impulse in the wire much the same as if the wire were stretched. In essence, it is a kind of "chemical" stretching of the wire, the result of which is the same as if the wire is "mechanically" stretched. That is, the wire is stimulated to carry the information to the brain, and the brain perceives this information from these pain carrying wires as a headache. An example of a vascular headache that is caused by inflammation of the blood vessels around the head is "temporal arteritis". This particular type headache is present in one or the other of the temples and can become so painful that simply touching the temple can cause severe pain. Fortunately, this type headache is relatively rare. It also only affects older patients, usually those in their 60's and older. Some of the previously mentioned types of migraines may be due to a combination of inflammation of the blood vessels as well as spasms of the blood vessels.

MISCELLANEOUS HEADACHES

We have now covered the causes of about 95% of all headaches. There are essentially only two more causes for headaches. Part of the remaining 5% of headaches is caused by abnormal impulses being generated within the pain carrying wires themselves without any external stimulation, unlike those that occur from compression of these wires by muscle spasms, (muscle contraction headaches) blood vessel spasms, (migraines) or from inflammation of blood vessels. It is generally unknown why these pain carrying wires suddenly begin sending signals to the brain without being irritated by some external cause. The headache that results from this cause is usually perceived as a sharp, shooting pain somewhere on the scalp that lasts only a second or two. It can occur only once in a while or can occur several times a day. It is when it becomes frequent in occurrence that a person usually seeks out treatment from a neurologist.

The rest of the remaining 5% of headaches is caused by compression of the pain carrying wires that are located in the lining of the sinuses and in the outer lining of the brain. By far, the greater number of these headaches is caused by compression of the lining of the sinuses than compression of the lining of the brain. The cause for this compression of the linings of the sinuses and the brain, which stretches the pain carrying wires contained within these linings that results in signals being sent to the brain and ultimately causes the headache is, in the case of the sinuses, fluid blockage of the sinuses, such as from a cold. In the case of the lining of the brain, masses within the brain itself push on the lining of the brain. This would include such things as tumors, collections of blood from a hemorrhage in the brain, cysts in the brain, and infections of the brain. Almost always, as mentioned in the preface of this book, a person will have other symptoms besides headache when the lining of the brain is compressed from a mass in the brain itself. This is why a neurologist is usually not too concerned about a tumor as the cause of a headache when there are no other neurologic symptoms, such as a change in personality, numbness on one side of the body, or weakness on one side.

It should be mentioned that the only part of the brain that actually has pain carrying wires is the lining of the brain. The brain itself cannot feel pain. It processes pain signals from other parts of the body such that a person is "aware" of pain in that particular part of the body, but does not send any pain signals from itself to itself, and therefore, cannot "feel" pain. The only way a tumor of the brain can cause a headache is if it becomes large enough to compress the lining of the brain, and to become large enough to do this, it almost certainly will compress some of the other parts of the brain itself to produce some of the associated symptoms mentioned above.

HEADACHES IN CHILDREN

Although children can get the same types of headaches as adults, as described above, headaches in children are more unusual and usually require more investigation into the underlying cause. Most muscle contraction headaches and vascular headaches are caused by stress. Children don't usually have the type of stress that triggers these headaches in adults, so when a child has frequent headaches, this is usually cause for concern.

In my experience, there are three causes for frequently occurring headaches in children.

First, children that have significant problems at home with interpersonal relationships, especially with their parents, seem to be more prone to frequent muscle contraction headaches. Unfortunately, these headaches don't seem to respond as readily to the usual medications used to treat these types of headaches in adults. Rather, the headaches are more likely to resolve when the problems at home resolve. As children get older, problems in school can be the most likely cause for frequent muscle contraction headaches.

Second, vascular headaches are very hereditary. Unfortunately, if a child's mother or father has severe migraines, there is a good chance that the child will have them too. They may occur more frequently or less frequently in the child than in the parent. They may also start at a younger age in the child than in the parent. I have seen children as young as 4 or 5 years old with vascular headaches, but never in a child this young who did not have a prominent family history of vascular headaches.

Third, seizures are frequently responsible for headaches in children. I would estimate that more than half of the children who have known seizure disorders have headaches, the frequency of which corresponds directly to the frequency of their seizures. The type headache that is associated with seizures is vascular in origin. The reason for these vascular headaches is easier to understand if one understands what happens in the brain during a seizure.

A seizure can be thought of as a "short" in the wiring of the brain. This short in the wiring of the brain can trigger an electrical storm that spreads to other parts of the brain, inappropriately activating thousands to millions of other wires in the brain. When this abnormally large number of wires becomes activated at the same time, this causes the patient to behave in an abnormal manner. He or she may lose consciousness, exhibit jerking type movements of the arms and legs, act zombie-like, or speak unintelligibly, depending on which part, and how much, of the brain is involved. The important part of all this, as far as the headaches associated with seizures are concerned, is that when there is so much electrical activity going on at one time in the wires of the brain, this requires a huge amount of energy to keep all these wires activated at the same time. In order to supply all this energy, which is continuously being carried from the blood vessels to the brain since the brain is incapable of storing energy within itself, the blood vessels have to dilate in order to hold more blood and hence, more glucose, which is the energy substance. As stated previously, when the blood vessels dilate, they stretch the pain carrying wires surrounding the blood vessels, which then send pain signals to the brain that the brain perceives as "headache". Therefore, either during the seizure, or after it is over, a patient may have a severe vascular headache.

Sometimes, when a patient has a seizure, he or she

has no outward signs that there is anything unusual going on within the brain. In these cases, it is not obvious to the patient that he or she is having a seizure, but when it is over, a severe vascular headache may still follow. At other times, seizures may occur while asleep, and go unnoticed except for a severe headache when awakening, either immediately after the seizure, or the next morning. These unnoticed, or "subclinical" seizures are the type that can oftentimes explain recurrent headaches in children who have never been diagnosed as having seizures. They can usually be diagnosed, however, by performing an electroencephalogram on the patient. (This test involves taping recording electrodes in several places on the patient's scalp to pick up any abnormal electrical signals being generated within the wires of the brain, such as from seizures, and will show the abnormal activity even when the patient is not aware that he or she is actually having a seizure at that particular time.)

As with adults, tumors, blood clots, and other space-occupying lesions in the brain are not common causes of headaches in children. In fact, these causes for headaches are even less likely to be seen in children than in adults.

TREATMENTS FOR HEADACHES

MUSCLE CONTRACTION HEADACHES

The treatment for muscle contraction headaches depends on the characteristics of the headache. If the headache has been present for a few hours, it would be treated differently than if it has been present continuously for several days of weeks. The cause for the muscle contraction headache, if able to be determined, also affects the type of treatment used to abolish the headache.

For muscle contraction headaches that have been present for up to a few hours, the treatment includes simple analgesics such as tylenol, aspirin, and other over-the-counter remedies. Occasionally, one of these short term headaches will not respond to over-the-counter remedies. In these cases, something a little stronger, such as one of the preparations of tylenol or aspirin mixed with caffeine and butalbital prescribed by a physician will usually work.

For muscle contraction headaches that last a few hours but then recur several times a week, or headaches that are continuous over several days or weeks, an analgesic alone will not work. In these cases, a "preventative" medication would need to be used. This preventative medication is one that would be taken every day, whether the patient has a headache at that particular time or not. Over a period of a few weeks, this medication will usually give resolution of the headaches. The types of medications that are used for abolishing these chronic muscle contraction headaches all fall under the heading of "anti-depressants". It should be mentioned that these are not used because the patient is thought to be depressed, necessarily, but rather because of the fact that they simply work. Like many secondary uses of medications, the use of anti-depressants for control of muscle contraction headaches was discovered by accident when it was noticed that while depressed patients who also had muscle contraction headaches were treated for their depression with the anti-depressants, their headaches were resolving too. Now these medications are used as much for control of muscle contraction headaches as for depression.

The way that the anti-depressant medications abolish muscle contraction headaches probably lies in the fact that they change the amount of various chemicals in the brain that control the passing of signals from one wire to another. If you will recall, muscle contraction headaches result from excess electrical activity in the brain which finds its way down through the brain to the spinal cord, and then out through the peripheral nerves to the muscles around the head and neck, causing these muscles to contract. The anti-depressants used to control muscle contraction headaches essentially "absorb" this excess electrical activity before it can filter down to the muscles around the head and neck to cause the typical muscle contraction headache. This is a relatively slow process that can take up to several weeks to work. However, results are usually seen within a week or so, in my experience.

Sometimes, the biggest problem with using anti-depressants to get rid of chronic muscle contraction headaches is convincing patients that the anti-depressants are not being given because the patient is thought to be depressed or "crazy". I have had occasional patients who have refused this treatment for that very reason.

The above treatment for chronic muscle contraction headaches works best for patients who have had some temporary cause for the headaches that has subsequently resolved even though the headache has continued because of the self perpetuating nature of muscle contraction headaches. For instance, the loss of a job can trigger a chronic muscle contraction headache that may continue even after another job has been found and the patient no longer is under the stress that this situation would have created. In these cases, a patient usually gets complete resolution of the chronic muscle contraction headache and can discontinue the medication after a month or so.

In cases where a patient has chronic stressors in his or her life, this treatment does not work as well, or, if it does help, the symptoms often return when the patient discontinues the medication. I have seen single mothers with five children aged 1 through 5 who live in small mobile homes with no visible means of support who have chronic muscle contraction headaches from all of these stressors that will never be relieved with the above treatment. There is no medical cure for headaches caused from these types of situations. The only cure in these cases is the one that results in changes in living conditions, and is better treated by social services departments than medications. Unfortunately, since it is sometimes not feasible to get rid of chronic stressors that cause continuous muscle contraction headaches, patients rely on pain killers, which as stated above, are only appropriate for occasional, or infrequent, muscle contraction headaches. This is because when analgesics, or pain killers, are taken frequently, they quickly lose their effectiveness, requiring the patient to take more of them at one time, or to seek a physician that doesn't mind giving stronger and stronger pain killers, most of which are very addictive. The resulting problem, drug addiction, is unfortunately not uncommon. In my experience, more than half of the patients who present with chronic muscle contraction headaches still have the stressors that caused these chronic headaches in the first place. These can be very difficult to treat unless, as stated above, the stressors can be eliminated. (Other alternative treatments for difficult to control headaches will be discussed below.)

VASCULAR HEADACHES

Treatment for vascular headaches involves simply relieving the cause for the stretching of the pain carrying wires that surround the blood vessels (arteries) located around the head. If the stretching of these blood vessels is caused from spasming of the blood vessels in the wide open position, then medications that control these spasms are indicated. These can be in the form of "preventive" type medications or "symptomatic" type medications. Preventive type medications are those that have to be taken on a daily basis to prevent the headaches from occurring. Symptomatic type pain relievers are used for immediate relief when the patient actually has a headache. Examples of preventive medications are the long acting forms of propranolol and nifedipine, which are usually taken every morning until the patient is headache free for a specific period of time. Symptomatic type pain relievers used for vascular headaches include the ergotamines and isometheptene, along with a few others. These are usually taken at the onset of a vascular headache and then repeated every half hour until either the headache is gone or until a certain number of them has been taken, such that if any more are taken, severe side effects can result. Usually, if a patient has more than one vascular headache in a month's time, a preventive type medication is indicated to keep the headaches away. For instance, if a patient has one vascular headache about every two or three months, it wouldn't make much sense, ordinarily, to take a medication every day to prevent this one headache when a symptomatic pain reliever may eliminate this infrequently occurring headache. I sometimes run across a patient who would rather take a medication every day than to have an incapacitating headache even as infrequently as once every six months. In these cases, the treatment regimen must be tailored to the specific needs of the patient.

For vascular headaches that are caused by stretching of the pain carrying wires by the swelling that occurs with inflammation of the blood vessel walls, a different class of medications is used for treatment. Anti-inflammatory medications can be used either as short term remedies or for long term control of these particular headaches. Steroids, such as prednisone, are also used for long term control of this type of vascular headache.

MISCELLANEOUS HEADACHES

Headaches caused by abnormal impulses being generated within the pain carrying wires themselves, without any external causes, are treated with medications that inhibit these abnormal impulses from being transmitted to the brain. Carbamazepine and clonazepam are the two most common medications used for this purpose. These are both preventive type treatments and are taken on a daily basis, ordinarily, until the patient has had no headaches for at least two weeks, at which point he or she can be tapered off the medication. Symptomatic type medications usually have no use in the treatment for these types of headaches since these headaches are fleeting, sharp, shooting pains that are gone in a second or two. (The only time they actually are treated with the above two medications is when they occur several times a day.)

Headaches caused from pressure on either the lining of the sinuses or the lining of the brain, both of which contain pain carrying wires susceptible to this pressure, are relieved with either treatments or medications that eliminate the pressure on these linings. In the case of pressure on the lining of the brain, this usually requires a surgical operation to remove the mass from within the brain. In the case of pressure on the linings of the sinuses, which is usually due to an excess of mucus in the sinus cavities, medications to reduce the mucus, such as cyproheptadine, are used.

There are many other types of treatments for the various types of headaches. Research is very active in looking for different medications for the treatment of headaches since this is such a common problem and has the potential of being very lucrative for a company that ultimately finds a new treatment. There are various medications that are given intravenously or into a muscle by injection that have shown some promise, especially for vascular headaches. For the most part, however, these are too cost prohibitive at the present time to be practical.

A patient's diet may have a lot to do with the frequency of his or her headaches. People who drink large amounts of caffeine are prone to caffeine withdrawal headaches, a type of vascular headache, when their intake of caffeine decreases for any reason on a particular day.

Some of the sugar substitutes and various other foods can trigger vascular headaches in susceptible individuals when taken in excess. The key word here is "excess". These various foods ordinarily do not cause headaches in most people when normal amounts are eaten.

There are several headache "clinics" around the country, with more of them springing up all the time. In some cases, they use exotic therapy regimens in attempting to rid the patient of his or her headaches. Other times, they use the standard treatment regimens, usually controlling the patient's diet and headache medications in a controlled environment in order to ultimately rid them of their headaches. In general, unless the patient's external stressors can be identified and ultimately eliminated, the headaches that cause a patient to eventually seek the treatment of a headache clinic will not resolve. Unfortunately, in my experience, headache clinics are usually not concerned with this fact. They have the potential for generating large amounts of income from desperate patients with chronic headaches and seem to capitalize on this. The generally poor long term results from treatment at a headache clinic attest to this.

In summary, 95% of headaches are due to muscle spasms and blood vessel spasms around the area of the head. Of these, 80% are due to muscle spasms and 15% are due to blood vessel spasms. The rest of the 5% of headaches are rare and of various causes.

Chapter 1

Chapter 2
CONFUSION

Confusion can mean different things to different people. To some, it may mean an inability to remember things. This is not accurate, however, because the inability to remember things really refers to memory loss. To others it may mean a feeling of dizziness. This also is not accurate. In fact, these two phenomena will be dealt with individually in later chapters. Confusion, to a neurologist, actually means an inability to form coherent thoughts. Along with this, a person who is confused is also unable to interpret external stimuli in an appropriate way. For instance, a confused person may pick up an orange and, because of its shape and size, mistakenly think it is a baseball and throw it rather than eat it. The sensory information, both from visually seeing the orange and from actually holding the orange, is not interpreted properly in the brain after this information is carried along the wires from the hand and from the eyes and finally reaches the brain. It is very important to remember that to use the term "confusion", the sensory information that is misinterpreted is done so in the brain itself and nowhere else. If a person injures one of the wires in the leg that carries information about the temperature of the foot, for example, then when this information travels from the area where the wire is damaged and finally reaches the brain, it may be misinterpreted because of the damage to the wire in the leg. This misinterpretation would not be labeled as "confusion" since the problem is in the leg, not the brain. Once one realizes that confusion occurs within the brain itself, it will be easier to understand how and why a person may exhibit a confused state.

Confusion occurs when the various parts of the brain are not able to communicate with each other. Remember, there are three types of wires in the entire nervous system: those that carry information towards the brain (sensory information, such as seeing, hearing, feeling, tasting, and smelling), those that carry information away from the brain (for moving muscles), and those that carry information "sideways", or, from one part of the brain to another part of the brain. It is these "sideways" nerves malfunctioning that produces "confusion". If one part of the brain is unable to communicate with another part of the brain, then appropriate decisions are not likely to result. This chapter will deal with diseases and other phenomena that affect the "sideways", or "communication", wires of the brain.

Some diseases of the nervous system can affect all three of the types of wires mentioned above and, in these cases, confusion is only a part of a much bigger picture of neurological impairment. This can usually be determined by doing a complete neurological examination on the patient, however.

We will deal first with diseases and phenomena that cause acute confusion, and then we will cover the diseases and phenomena that cause chronic confusion.

ACUTE CONFUSION

MEDICATIONS AND DRUGS

The most common cause of acute confusion without other neurological impairment is the effects of medications on the brain. If one looks in the Physician's Desk Reference (PDR), which lists all of the various medications, their effects on the body, and their side effects, he or she would see that most medications may cause confusion as a side effect. If a person is on more than one medication, the chances of confusion resulting are increased. In my experience, over 90% of the patients that I am asked to see in consultation because of acute confusion are determined to be confused because of a problem with a medication, either because a new medication was recently started, or because the patient is receiving to much of a particular medication.

The chemicals that are contained within the brain and cause the brain to function in a normal manner are under very rigid control. In fact, there is a barrier between the brain and the rest of the body that prevents most substances from even getting into the brain by way of the blood which allows the brain to maintain this rigid control. Many medications are able to breach this barrier and find their way into the brain. This upsets the fine tuned control of the electrical impulses being generated within the wires of the brain. When information carried in these wires from one part of the brain to another part of the brain is interfered with, the wires may carry wrong information, or they may carry the information to the wrong place in the brain. The result is seen as "confusion".

There are other substances that are not usually thought of as "medications" which, nevertheless, affect the functioning of the brain in such a way that acute confusion is the result. Alcohol is probably the most common substance that affects the brain in this way. Alcohol very easily passes through the barrier that prevents most substances from entering the brain. Once the alcohol is in contact with the brain itself, it prevents information from being carried from one wire to another, somewhat like turning off the switch on a lamp. Other "drugs", such as the various narcotics, amphetamines, and cocaine, also affect the brain by interfering with the transmission of information across the wires from one place to another within the brain itself. When a patient arrives in an emergency room in a confused state, he or she will usually be checked for the presence of "drugs", such as those mentioned above, as a cause for the acute confusion.

The brain relies on a constant supply of sugar from the blood (in the form of glucose) for energy to keep the wires that make up the brain working as intended. This sugar is carried to the brain continuously, dissolved in the blood. If, for some reason, the concentration of sugar in the blood drops, then a person may become acutely confused as a first sign of this drop in blood sugar. "Confusion" results as the primary symptom because the communication wires of the brain that carry information from one part of the brain to another are more susceptible to acute decreases of sugar in the blood than the wires that carry information towards or away from the brain. (If the concentration of sugar in the blood continues to fall, then these other two types of information carrying wires will eventually be affected too.) If a patient arrives in the emergency room in a confused state, the patient's glucose level in the blood is also checked for a possible cause of his or her confusion. Normally, people will not have this type of a problem unless they are diabetic and have taken too much insulin, which helps to remove glucose from the blood and transfers it into the cells of the body where it is used for energy.

BLOOD FLOW TO THE BRAIN

A less common cause for acute confusion is a decrease in the blood flow to the brain. Since the brain relies on a constant stream of nutrients (in the form of glucose dissolved in the blood) for its energy source, anything that interferes with the normal flow of blood to the brain will have an effect on the delivery of the glucose in the blood to the brain, which can cause confusion as a first symptom of something wrong within the brain.

Heart arrhythmias are the most common causes of acute changes in the blood flow to the brain. The heart is designed to beat in an orderly fashion such that the blood is squeezed out of the heart in a wavelike manner. If a person suddenly develops palpitations or a fluttering of the heart, the blood is not pumped out of the heart smoothly, and this results in less blood leaving the heart. If less blood leaves the heart, then less blood arrives at the brain. If these heart arrhythmias last for longer than 5 or 6 seconds, acute confusion may result. Sometimes, it may take a few hours for the brain to recover from this acute lack of nutrients, and the patient may remain acutely confused for these few hours. Oftentimes, a person will give a history of palpitations prior to becoming confused, but sometimes the patient is unaware that this phenomenon is taking place. This, of course, makes it more difficult to determine the cause of the acute confusion. There are various monitoring devices for the heart that can record these spells, but if the patient only has a spell very infrequently, then the chances of documenting one with these devices are very poor.

Another way that the flow of blood to the brain can be altered, resulting in acute confusion, is through spasms of the blood vessels that carry the blood to the brain. These blood vessel spasms can result in marked constriction of the blood vessels which impedes the flow of blood to the brain, resulting in acute confusion. In people who have a history of high blood pressure, this is sometimes referred to as a "hypertensive crisis". Some types of vascular headaches can cause vascular spasms severe enough to result in acute confusion. (It should be mentioned that we are referring to a matter of degree of impairment of blood flow resulting in acute confusion. That is, if the impairment of blood flow is mild, or for a shorter period of time, acute confusion may result. If the impairment of blood flow is more severe, or for a longer period of time, the patient may actually lose consciousness. This will be dealt with in the chapter on "blackouts".)

Acute confusion may result from a loss of blood, such as from a bleeding ulcer in the stomach or in the intestines. In these cases, the communication wires of the brain, which are the first wires to become affected, do not get enough nutrients from the blood flow to the brain because there is not enough blood to keep the pressure up high enough to supply the brain with enough glucose.

SENSORY DEPRIVATION

The brain, while awake, depends on a constant source of input from the sensory wires, which carry information towards the brain from the outlying areas of the body. As already mentioned, this can be in the form of visual, audio, touch, smell, or taste information. The brain constantly processes this incoming information in order to stay active. When there is not enough outside information available for the brain to process while the person is awake, or when the sensory modalities themselves are impaired, such as from loss of vision or loss of hearing, it will "create" its own "sensory" information by sending impulses back and forth between the communication wires within the brain. When this occurs, the person appears acutely confused because he or she is not reacting to external sensory stimuli in an appropriate manner. Oftentimes, when a patient who has mildly impaired hearing or vision is confined in a hospital, or other unfamiliar surroundings, he or she will often become acutely confused when it becomes dark outside, and sensory input to the brain is decreased even more. This phenomenon occurs so commonly in hospitals that it has been given the name, "sundowning". Sensory deprivation chambers produce acute confusion for the same reasons as described above.

CHRONIC CONFUSION

Chronic confusion results from permanent or continuing impairment of the communication wires of the brain. This can occur because of chronic use of medications or drugs that affect the communication wires of the brain, from chronic decrease in the blood flow to the brain, or from predetermined (genetic) death of the communication wires of the brain.

MEDICATIONS AND DRUGS

There are few medications that will cause permanent confusion. Usually, once the medication is discontinued, the confusion resolves. However, some people must remain on a medication that may cause confusion as a side effect because of the greater risk to their survival if they discontinue the medication. For all practical purposes, in these cases, a person has what we can call "chronic confusion". Of course, if a person remained confused all the time with one of these types of medications, it probably wouldn't make sense to use it in spite of its life preserving qualities, since the person's quality of life in the chronically confused state wouldn't be much of a life at all. The chronic confusion with these medications refers to the fact that the person who uses the medication may be confused at certain times of the day (usually in the evening), but not all the time. More often, chronic confusion results from continuous use of non-prescribed medications, or drugs.

The most commonly used drug that results in chronic confusion is alcohol. When used excessively over a long period of time, it can permanently damage the communication wires in the brain such that a person may be confused even when not acutely intoxicated.

Although it is not usually thought of as a typical "medication", radiation treatments that are given to destroy cancer cells can be thought of as a type of medication. When these treatments are given for cancers that occur in the brain, they can destroy the cells in the brain that transfer the nutrients, such as glucose, from the blood to the wires in the brain where they are used for energy. When this occurs, the nutrients are not able to get into the wires where they are needed and a chronic state of confusion can result.

BLOOD FLOW TO THE BRAIN

Chronic changes in the supply of blood to the brain can result in chronic confusion. Specifically, decreases in the flow of blood to the brain are what cause the chronic confusion. This can occur either because of chronic constriction of the blood vessels (vascular spasms), or a chronically low volume of blood.

Hypertension refers to chronically constricted blood vessels. In the brain, one of the most sensitive areas to this chronically decreased supply of blood and its associated nutrients is the communication wires. After several years of being deprived of an adequate supply of nutrients, these wires slowly begin dying, and the person becomes chronically confused. An even more prominent cause of chronic confusion from these chronically constricted blood vessels is the eventual closing up of these blood vessels completely. When a blood vessel is constantly in the constricted state, it builds up a thicker muscle in its wall. As this muscle gets thicker and thicker, the opening in the center of the blood vessel gets smaller and smaller until finally, the opening in the center is completely closed off. When blood can no longer flow through the blood vessel, all the parts of the brain that that particular blood vessel supplies die. This is called a "stroke". The blood vessels being referred to, in this case, are very tiny ones, and only supply a very tiny area of the brain with blood. The person in whom this phenomenon occurs will not even be aware that a stroke has occurred. With time, however, the person may become more and more confused as more and more of these tiny strokes occur. Remember, the communication wires of the brain are among the most susceptible to these tiny strokes because of the way the architecture of the blood vessel system (vascular system) is laid out in the brain. The communication wires of the brain have one of the poorest blood supplies and, because of this, are among the first to be affected by decreases in the amount of blood being delivered to the brain. The chronic confusion that results from more and more of these tiny strokes occurring in the communication areas of the brain contributes to a phenomenon called "multi-infarct dementia". This is the most common cause of dementia in the elderly. Eventually, if one lives long enough, he or she will ultimately suffer from this process because, even if a person does not have chronically constricted blood vessels, such as from high blood pressure (hypertension), the blood vessels will still form deposits on the walls, much like the water pipes in a house as it ages, that will eventually cause the blood vessel to close up completely. The smaller the blood vessel is in the first place, the sooner it will close up. And since the smallest blood vessels in the brain are in the communication areas, multi-infarct dementia is what appears first from this phenomenon. (These tiny strokes in the smallest blood vessels don't usually cause paralysis because the blood vessels that supply the wires going from the brain to the muscles are mostly larger. If one of the larger blood vessels that supplies nutrients to the wires that carry information from the brain to the muscles closes up for any reason, then what we usually think of as a "stroke", with paralysis, occurs. This will be dealt with later in the chapter on "weakness".)

GENETIC CAUSES OF CHRONIC CONFUSION

The most common cause of chronic confusion that is of genetic origin is Alzheimer's disease. Much research is being done on this particular disease in order to find a cure, or at least a treatment, for it. The abnormality in the genetic material that causes Alzeimer's disease is being identified. Researchers already know which chromosome is involved with the abnormality that causes this disease. It is also known why this disease occurs. That is, there is a defect in the way that various chemicals are broken down within the brain cells such that there is a break in the sequence of events that ultimately converts these chemicals from one form to another. This causes a buildup of the one chemical that cannot be converted properly to the next chemical in the sequence of events within the brain cell involved. The accumulation of this chemical within that brain cell eventually kills the cell. For example, if chemical A is converted to chemical B, and chemical B is converted to chemical C, but there is a defect that prevents chemical B from being converted to chemical C, then there will be a buildup of chemical B in the cell as more and more of chemical A is converted to chemical B. As chemical B fills up the cell, the usual workings of the cell become impaired because of all the crowding and the cell dies. In Alzheimer's disease, as you may have guessed by now, this process resulting in cell death occurs in large part in the communication wires of the brain, which results in the chronic confusion that results from this disease. There are other less abundant genetic diseases that cause chronic confusion, such as Huntington's disease, well known because of its appearance in the family of the singer, Woody Guthrie. Although this particular disease affects different groups of communication wires than Alzheimer's disease, the process is essentially the same as described above.

In summary, it is important to remember that confusion is associated with problems in the communication wires of the brain. If only the other two types of wires in the nervous system are involved in some particular disease process (those that carry information towards the brain and those that carry information away from the brain), then sensory loss or weakness may result, but not confusion. The most common cause of confusion is medications that a person may be taking.

Chapter 2

Chapter 3
MEMORY LOSS

Memory is probably the most interesting and intriguing phenomenon of the nervous system. Its sole purpose is to enable us to retain information. Without memory, we would not even know who we are. We also would not be able to form relationships with others, our personalities would be very bland, to say the least, and probably most important, we would be unable to learn.

We have three types of memory, classified by length of time that they enable us to retain information. They are immediate, recent, and remote memories. In order to understand how our memories can fail, it is first necessary to understand how our three memory systems work. Although there is still some disagreement on the actual mechanism of memory, the following explanations are generally accepted as the way our three memory systems work.

IMMEDIATE MEMORY

Our immediate memory allows us to remember infor-

mation that we have just obtained, either by hearing it, seeing it, feeling it, smelling it, or tasting it. When we look up
a phone number and then remember it long enough to dial
it without writing it down, this involves our immediate
memory. Immediate memory is retained only for a very
short period of time, and then is lost forever, unless the
information is important enough to be transferred into one
of the longer-term memory systems.

Immediate memory consists of an electrical circuit
that is set up in the deeper parts of the brain by incoming
information. It travels around this area of the brain in a circular fashion until it finally fizzles out, which is when the
memory for this particular information is lost forever. The
key to understanding how immediate memory works is to
remember that all information that reaches the brain from
our five senses is in the form of electrical impulses, as this
is the only type of medium that the brain can use for processing information. As long as this electrical information
is traveling on the wires within the brain, the information
contained on these wires is accessible by other parts of the
brain to use for whatever purpose the brain wishes. For
instance, using the example of dialing a new phone number when the number is remembered by looking it up in the
phone book but not writing it down, the brain channels this
information that is traveling in a circular fashion in the
wires of the deeper parts of the brain to the part of the brain
that controls finger movements such that a person's fingers
will dial the number on the phone that corresponds to the
number that is contained within the continuous electrical
circuit that was set up in the deeper part of the brain on the
immediate memory circuit.

It was mentioned above that the circuit that contains
immediate memory information eventually "fizzles" out.
This is not entirely true. What actually happens is that new
information is continually coming into the deeper areas of
the brain that contain the wires used for these circuits, and

this new information "bumps" the old information out of the circuit. The old information is then lost forever. When we repeat information over and over to ourselves in order to remember it long enough to use the information before we forget it, we are actually renewing the information on the immediate memory circuits before it can be replaced by other new information that is continually being sent from the five senses to the information processing area of this deeper part of the brain. This same process of "bumping" occurs when someone interrupts us while we are trying to perform some immediate memory related task. We forget what we were trying to remember when the person talks to us, unless we concentrate on what we were trying to remember before we were interrupted. In this case, the word "concentrate" means to repeat the previous information over and over to ourselves so that it continuously replaces onto the immediate memory circuits the incoming information from the person's voice who interrupted us. For instance, if you repeat a phone number over and over while someone is talking to you, you are more likely to remember it than if you say it once, then listen to the person who is talking to you, then try to remember it. These circuits in the deeper brain for immediate memory are very limited in number. This is why we can only take in a relatively small amount of information at one time.

The most important thing to remember about immediate memory, so that it will be easier to understand why this memory system may fail, is that it is dynamic, or continuously in motion. That is, there is continuous electrical activity circulating in the deeper part of the brain in order for the immediate memory to work. Once this electrical activity stops, then immediate memory stops also at that instant. Immediate memory systems do not "store" any information.

To summarize, sensory information travels from the peripheral nerves (wires) to the deeper part of the brain. In this part of the brain, it travels in a self perpetuating circular pathway from one immediate memory wire to another, over and over again, over the same wires, until new sensory information arrives and replaces this information on the immediate memory wires. While this information is circulating through the immediate memory cycle, the higher brain centers can either extract the information and use it in some way, or can ignore it and let it be abolished (forgotten) when new information replaces it on the immediate memory cycle. All information from the immediate memory system that is not used in some way by the higher brain centers is lost forever because the immediate memory system itself has no way of storing any information.

REMOTE MEMORY

Remote memory is what we usually think about when we refer to our "memory". It consists of stored information only, unlike the immediate memory system, which has no stored information. The remote memory system is a permanent memory system. In order to understand how the remote memory system works, it is important to again remember that the brain functions only as a result of the interactions between the living wires that are contained within it. From about the age of 6 or 7, the total number of wires in the brain does not change. What does change, and what is responsible for giving us each our own individual personalities, emotions, and abilities for learning new information is the number of branches and different connections to other wires that each individual wire contains.

If one thinks of the wires as the trunks of trees that are very close to one another, with all the branches in the wires like the branches of trees, all intertwined with the branches of the neighboring trees, the concept will be easier to grasp. In the case of the wires and their branches in the brain, however, there is an important difference. That is, the branches of the wires in the brain actually make electrical connections with other branches in their immediate vicinities. They can connect to branches from other wires, branches from their own wires, or even to themselves by doubling back upon themselves. The particular connection that is made by one individual branch of a wire may code for one particular memory, such as a person's age, for example. The number of branches that can grow off a wire within the brain, and the number of branches this particular branch can ultimately choose to connect with, are essentially unlimited. This is why we can store so much information in our remote memory systems.

One might wonder what the actual stored substance of a particular memory is in the brain. Again, this may be a difficult concept to understand unless one continues to remember that everything the brain is and does is dictated by the current that travels through the various wires that make up the brain. If current happens to travel through the branch of the wire mentioned above that codes for a person's age, he or she will immediately be conscious of this. If current travels through one of the branches of a wire in the brain that codes for some event that happened when the person was twenty years younger, he or she will immediately become conscious of this particular event. As can be seen, remote memory is "stored" as individual branches of the wires of the brain, along with the connections they may make to other wires, or branches of other wires. That is, to form a new permanent memory, one of the wires of the brain must sprout a new branch or make a new connection. Every time an electric current passes through this new branch, the person will be consciously aware of the same event that occurred when that particular branch was formed. Although this may seem to be a crude way to form a remote memory system, it is essentially unlimited in its ability to form new memories. Unfortunately, it is prone to logistics problems, the haphazard way in which the branches are formed on the wires of the brain making retrieval of information from remote memory very difficult at times. This will be explained below.

The deeper parts of the brain have many functions. One of these functions is to keep a continuous current flowing in the brain, even when we are not actively processing sensory information, such as when we are asleep. This can be compared to leaving a car engine idling in neutral while waiting at a railroad crossing. As long as we are alive, there is current flowing through some part of our brain. When we try to remember some event that happened in the past, we are actually trying to direct this flow of current in our brain towards the particular branch of the wire in our remote memory system that codes for that event. If the event we are trying to remember was not a significant one, it may have been coded on a distant branch that is far from the mainstream, somewhat like trying to find a house off the beaten path up a winding backwoods road, as opposed to locating a gas station right off the interstate. This differs from a computer memory, in which all information is essentially equally retrievable.

Our remote memory system is prone to problems. There are at least two reasons for this. First, even though current may be directed to the general area of a memory that is trying to be retrieved, it may not reach the exact area of intended retrieval and another memory may be retrieved instead, or no memory at all. Second, because the brain is "plastic", or relatively easily changed structurally, some of the branches of the wires that code for various memories may change their shapes or connections over time, especially if not retrieved very often, such that the memory is not accurate any longer, or may even disappear completely.

Occasionally, various memories will be associated with other memories. For instance, certain fragrances can be associated with certain people. When one smells that particular fragrance, a mental picture of a specific person may be formed. This is most likely because when the permanent memory of this particular fragrance was being formed as a branch of one of the wires in the brain, the memory of the person it was associated with was formed in close proximity to this branch. Then, whenever that fragrance is smelled, the electrical impulse generated in the brain by the fragrance upon the smell receptors in the nose is directed to the memory of the fragrance in the remote memory system of the brain and, because of the close location of the memory of the person with the memory of the fragrance, the current also spreads to that branch as well, resulting in not only a recollection of the fragrance, but also of the person with whom it was associated. When we use association techniques to improve our memories, we are probably applying this same principle. That is, we are using more than one memory branch to attract electrical current to a particular area of the remote memory system for recall of a particular memory in that area. It is not always easy to direct the electrical current in the brain to a particular area, but with more memory branches in one area "calling" the current, it is more likely to find its way to that particular area. Once it is in that area, it is easier for the current to "find" the memory being recalled.

There have been experiments done by neurosurgeons where an electric probe is used to touch various parts of an exposed brain while the patient is awake, stimulating that particular part of the brain with an electric current. Some patients reported "hearing" melodies from songs they had not heard for several years when the part of the brain was stimulated that contained the remote memory branches that coded for those particular songs when the memories were formed years before.

To summarize the remote memory system, it is contained as a system of branches of some of the wires in the brain that, when an electric current passes along a particular one of these memory branches, causes a person to have a conscious recollection of an event just as when that particular event originally occurred.

RECENT MEMORY

The mechanism of recent memory includes some of the workings of both immediate and remote memory. It is thought to be located in the temporal lobes of the brain, an area that is more or less between the deeper parts of the brain where immediate memory is located and the higher parts of the brain where remote memory is located. This memory system can record information for up to a few days, and then it is either lost forever or transferred into remote memory where it will last indefinitely. It can be thought of as the "middleman" in our memory system. Electrical impulses are diverted from the circular system of immediate memory to the recent memory areas where it causes changes in the branches of the wires of the brain. These changes in the recent memory branches occur faster than the changes in the remote memory branches, but what they gain in speed they lose in permanence. This works out nicely, though, because it allows us to quickly remove important sensory information from immediate memory before more incoming sensory information replaces it on the immediate memory circuits and stores it long enough to decide whether we want to keep it forever or forget it.

The recent memory system is constantly forming new memory branches while breaking down older ones. This prevents the recent memory area from having to expand in size.

To summarize the relationship of the three memory systems before going into how these systems fail, the immediate memory is electrical impulses only. As long as the current continues to flow in the circular pattern through the immediate memory, we are aware of the sensory information it contains. Recent memory contains both electrical circuits, like the ones in immediate memory, and branches on the wires in this area of the brain, each of which contains coded memories in the way that the branches are formed and in the connections that they make with other branches near them. These branches are not permanent and are replaced every few days with new memory branches. Remote memory is stored as branches of the wires in the brain's remote memory areas. These are permanent branches and probably take a day or two to form. When an electric current passes through a memory branch, the person becomes immediately conscious of the particular memory that is encoded by that branch.

FAILURE OF THE MEMORY SYSTEM

Since each memory system has its own peculiar way of functioning, then it is conceivable that a disease state could affect any one of the three systems individually. Of course, some diseases can, and do, affect all three memory systems at the same time.

REMOTE MEMORY LOSS

In my experience, about 80% of the patients that I am asked to see because of a complaint of "memory loss" are not actually suffering from a "loss" of memory but, rather, an inability to "recall" particular memories. Another way of stating this inability to recall is a lack of "concentration". This can affect any of the three memory systems, but is usually more associated with recent memory. Concentration is the act of directing the generator current that is always present in the brainstem (like a car that is idling in neutral at a railroad crossing) towards a particular memory branch, either in recent or remote memory areas, in order to bring that particular memory into consciousness by electrical stimulation. The most common cause of lack of concentration is preoccupation with something. For instance, if someone is worried about a relative that may be very sick in the hospital, his or her current generator is actively sending electrical current to the memories in the recent and remote memory systems that pertain to the sick person, such as memories of the emotional attachment to the sick person and images of the sick person. Because of this directing of the generator current to memories related to the sick person, other memories are not able to be recalled as easily. (This is what is meant by the term "preoccupied".) Also, along the same line, when new information coming from the five senses reaches the immediate memory circuits in the deeper areas of the brain, it is quickly "bumped" out of the circuit by sensory information that pertains to the sick person because, at that particular time, information about the sick person is considered to be the most important by the brain.

As one can see, the above cause of "memory loss" is not really due to an actual "disease" of the nervous system. It is due to external influences upon the brain, and resolves when the external influences are resolved.

Occasionally, there may be internal causes for a lack of concentration that a person may interpret as a memory loss. These internal causes are due to an abnormally low amount of one or more of the various chemicals (transmitters) that allow the electric current in the wires of the brain to jump from one wire to the next in any given sequence. There are several reasons why these transmitter chemicals might be low. For instance, not getting enough vitamins may affect the levels, various hormones can affect the levels, and low levels of these chemicals can be hereditary in origin. Depression without any obvious external cause is probably the most classic example of abnormal levels of chemical transmitters.

The remaining 20% of patients seen in my practice

who complain of memory loss actually have a true memory loss rather than a lack of concentration. Most of the people suffering from a true memory loss are advanced in age and either have one of the Alzheimer-like diseases or multi infarct dementia.

The Alzheimer diseases are caused by an accumulation of unusable protein products in the actual wires of the brain that ultimately prevents the wires from functioning as they are intended. No one knows for sure why this protein "junk" is allowed to accumulate within the wires, but, as stated in the previous chapter, it is thought to be due to a loss of ability to break down the various nutrients taken into the wire for its ongoing maintenance and for production of energy for transmitting current along the wire. This defect is felt to be due to a predetermined genetic defect. However, it may also be due to a "wearing out" of the cell with age, such that it can no longer process chemicals adequately.

Among the first wires affected in the brain by the Alzheimer's diseases are those that deal with memory, and only much later are the wires that deal with movement affected. This is why people with Alzheimer's disease usually are not impaired in their ability to walk or hold a fork to eat, even though they may be unable to carry on an intelligent conversation any longer. It is not known why the memory wires are among the first involved in this process, but we do know that as the process continues, it eventually involves most of the various wires of the brain, including the wires for moving the arms and legs.

There is no cure for the Alzheimer diseases, but there have been some medications developed purported to slow down the process. In my experience, none of these have proven to be effective, however, and are not worth mentioning.

Multi-infarct dementia is caused by a decreased blood flow to the brain over a long period of time. This can be due to atherosclerosis, which is a narrowing of the opening in the interior of the blood vessels from the normal aging process, or from chronic high blood pressure. This type of dementia can also occur when the heart is not strong enough to pump enough blood to the brain over a long period of time.

The memory wires of the brain are susceptible to changes in the delivery of blood to the brain because they have one of the poorest blood supplies of any part of the brain. Anything that affects the blood supply to the brain, especially over a long period of time, will usually permanently affect the memory system.

Multi-infarct dementia will eventually affect all of us, if we live long enough. This is because, as stated in the previous chapter on confusion, it can be due to the normal aging process, which includes a filling up of the blood vessels with "junk" as we age that will ultimately cause a decreased amount of blood arriving at the memory areas of the brain. When the blood supply finally is so diminished that it ceases flowing, a tiny infarct, or dead area of the brain, results in the area of the brain that that blood vessel supplied. When many of these tiny little dead areas exist over a long period of time, we can recognize a noticeable decline in an ability to remember things, hence the name, "multi-infarct" dementia. (It should be mentioned that these tiny infarcts, or strokes, go unnoticed individually because they involve very tiny blood vessels, and therefore, very tiny parts of the brain. This is unlike what we usually think of as a stroke where a large blood vessel becomes blocked, usually by a blood clot, and the patient has a noticeable loss of some function, such as paralysis on one side. Since a larger blood vessel is involved, a larger part of the brain dies.)

The usual treatment for multi-infarct dementia is blood thinners, such as aspirin or warfarin. The theory behind the use of blood thinners is that if the blood is made thinner, it can flow through the smaller openings in the tiny blood vessels more easily. This treatment does seem to slow down the process.

Some other causes of true memory loss are more rare and involve the ingestion of drugs or toxins. Alcohol is probably the most common drug that can result in memory loss over an extended period of time. Again, the wires of the brain with the poorest blood supply seem to be the ones that are most affected by drugs and toxins over a prolonged period of time with frequent ingestion, as is the case with alcoholics. This may be because these areas of the brain are not able to clear out the drug as fast as the areas that have a better blood flow through them which results in the drug exerting its toxic influence on these areas of the brain for relatively longer periods of time.

Even rarer than drugs or toxins as a cause for real memory loss are genetic disorders. These disorders seem to work similar to the Alzheimer type diseases. That is, they usually involve an accumulation of protein molecules in the wires of the memory system of the brain that eventually cause the death of those wires because of an inability to process these proteins so that they can be eliminated, ultimately. Down's syndrome is one of the most common genetic disorders that causes memory loss in this way. Usually, by the time someone with Down's syndrome reaches the age of thirty, he or she has begun to exhibit signs of dementia.

RECENT AND IMMEDIATE MEMORY LOSS

The most common cause of immediate or recent memory loss is trauma to the head. This doesn't actually have to involve physical contact between the head and another object, but can result even from a whiplash type injury where the head doesn't hit anything. What does have to occur, however, is at least a brief loss of consciousness. When a person loses consciousness, the electric memory circuit in the immediate memory system stops. Any events that were being processed for eventual storage into remote memory are lost forever. This is why a person has amnesia for, or can't remember, events that occurred for several minutes just prior to losing consciousness. These events are still in immediate memory, and when this circuit is temporarily turned off, they are abolished. Once the person regains consciousness, it takes some time for the brain to start up the immediate memory circuits again, which results in an inability to form an immediate memory for up to several days, depending on how long the person was unconscious.

Since recent memory is constantly dependent upon the immediate memory system for input, it too is affected by a loss of consciousness. Any information that is in the process of being stored in the recent memory system is lost forever when the electrical circuits are interrupted. This can prolong the amount of time that a person is unable to form permanent memories after he or she awakens from a period of loss of consciousness.

A lack of certain vitamins or other essential nutrients can cause failures in the immediate or recent memory systems.

An interesting phenomenon that occurs in people who are chronic alcoholics who don't eat well enough to maintain an adequate supply of thiamine in their brains is that they are unable to form new memories because of the isolated effect of lack of thiamine on their immediate memory system. If asked to remember something for much longer than a few seconds, they are unable to do so. Their remote memories remain intact, and they can recall events from their remote memories, but they can no longer put any new memories into their remote memories. This is called Korsakoff's syndrome.

Selective memory loss occurs when the brain actively

prevents certain memories from being recalled. When the current generator attempts to send an electrical signal to one of the branches in the recent or remote memory area of the brain, it is blocked by a stronger electric current coming from another part of the brain (usually one of the emotional centers) that steers the current off down another wire instead. For instance, if a person witnesses a brutal murder, he or she will form a permanent memory of this event in the remote memory system. He or she will also form a permanent memory in the emotional memory of the brain as well. This will not be a memory of the actual event but a memory of the fear that was associated with the event. When the memory for the event is attempted to be recalled by sending an electric current from the current generator in the deeper parts of the brain towards the wire that contains this memory branch, it also sends a current to the memory branch that was formed at the same time in the emotional memory center of the remote memory system. The current probably arrives at the emotional memory system first before it reaches the actual event as stored in the remote memory system, and is either diverted or canceled by the emotional memory branch before it can activate the memory of the event in the remote memory system. This may explain why a person may become frightened when a particularly upsetting event is mentioned to him or her, but has no actual recall of the event. That is, the sensory information about the event that the person hears stimulates the current generator to send an electric impulse towards both the emotional and actual memory of the event in the remote memory system but it arrives at the emotional memory system first, which makes the person feel frightened, but then the emotional memory system stops the impulse from reaching the actual memory of the event and the person is unaware of why he or she is frightened. Sodium pentothal (truth serum) has its effect on the current carrying capacity of the wires of the brain and probably works by interrupting the current from the emotional memory areas so that it is not diverted away from the actual memory of a particularly frightening event, such that it can be recalled once the person is given this drug.

In summary, the three different memory systems work in different ways that make them singly susceptible to various diseases resulting in various types of memory loss. About 80% of people who complain of memory loss don't actually have a loss of memory, but rather, a lack of concentration that makes it difficult to recall a memory.

Chapter 4
DIZZINESS

Everyone has been dizzy at one time or another. The most difficult thing about diagnosing the cause of dizziness is first determining what a person means when he or she refers to feeling "dizzy".

There are two types of dizziness. One type is a lightheaded feeling, and the second type refers to a feeling of a spinning sensation, which is called vertigo. The symptoms of these two types of dizziness are very different, but sometimes it is difficult for a person to describe which type of dizziness is being experienced. Vertigo can occur in any position, including lying down, sitting up, or standing. Lightheadedness usually only occurs in going from the lying to sitting or standing position, or while remaining in the standing position for a period of time. We will first discuss vertigo and its causes, and then we will discuss lightheadedness and its causes.

VERTIGO

An attack of vertigo can occur at any age but is usually more commonly seen as a person ages, the reason for which will become evident soon.

There are only two areas in the entire body that can be responsible for an attack of vertigo. In order to understand why vertigo occurs, it is first necessary to understand the normal function of the two areas involved. The first area is located in the inner ear on both sides and involves the semi-circular canals.

The semi-circular canals consist of three ring-like structures at about 45 degree angles from each other, such that one is parallel to the ground, one is perpendicular to the ground, and the third is at an angle half way in between these two. These three canals are filled with fluid and have tiny nerve endings protruding into the fluid-filled spaces through the walls of the canals. There are also tiny, free floating "rocks" contained within these semi-circular canals that actually roll across the nerve endings when a person moves his or her head. (These nerve endings fall under the category of mechanoreceptors because they send sensory information to the brain in response to movement of the individual nerve endings.) When a person moves his or her head in a straight forward manner, the rock in the semi-circular canal that is parallel to the ground moves across the nerve endings protruding into that canal, which causes these nerves to carry sensory information to the brain telling it that the body is moving in a foreward manner. If a person moves upwards or downwards, the nerve endings in the semi-circular canal perpendicular to the ground become stimulated by the rock in that canal moving up or down across the nerve endings, which then carry sensory information to the brain that lets the brain know that the body is moving upwards or downwards. Combinations of movements of the body stimulate combinations of movements of the various rocks across the nerve endings in the three semi-circular canals to let the brain know at every instant where the body is in space at that particular time.

One would think that a sophisticated system such as described above would be fairly large in size, but this is not the case. Each semi-circular canal is only about one- fourth inch in diameter, and is embedded in the bone behind the actual hearing apparatus on each side of the head.

The second area that can be involved when a person has an attack of vertigo is in the group of wires that carry the information from the semi-circular canals to the higher brain centers. After the wires leave the area within the semi-circular canals, they travel in a bundle to the brain-stem where they cross over to the other side of the brain-stem, then travel up to the higher areas of the brain where they interact with either the communication wires of the brain or with the memory areas of the brain to effect some reaction to the movement of the body. For instance, if a person begins falling to one side, the rocks in the semi-circular canals will move, stimulating the nerve endings, which then send an electric current through the bundle of wires to the brainstem, then up to the higher areas of the brain where the electric current is processed. The brain then acts on all this sensory information by sending an impulse from the brain to the spinal cord, and then to the leg, telling it to move in order to brace the person so that he or she doesn't fall. (Remember, all information leaving the brain is for the purpose of moving muscles.)

Hopefully, it is starting to become a little clearer that the areas of the brain that, when they fail, cause vertigo are normally used for the purpose of maintaining our balance.

Over 90% of spells of vertigo are caused by a malfunction in the semi-circular canals. One of the most common malfunctions is caused by viral infections such as from a cold or flu. It is thought that the viruses somehow cause the pressure of the fluid in the semi-circular canals to increase or decrease in such a way that it affects the nerve endings contained within the canals such that they send erroneous sensory information to the brain for processing because the left and right side semi-circular canals are not in agreement. When the information coming from the right side does not agree exactly with the left side, vertigo results. This is because the brain is receiving conflicting information about where the body is in space any time a movement is made. In order to stop the vertigo, a person will try to remain perfectly still to keep the rocks in the semi-circular canals from rolling around and stimulating the right and left sides differently. (Nausea is oftentimes associated with vertigo and this is thought to be due to the constant attempts by the brain to synchronize the differing sensory information that is arriving at the brain from the right and left semi-circular canals. This can be thought of as a type of "overload" of sensory electrical current in the brain, and is somewhat like the nausea that results from being on a boat that is constantly moving, which also presents an overload of sensory information from the semi-circular canals to the brain from the rocks rolling around in the semi-circular canals continuously with this constant movement. The nausea center is located near the balance center, and when the balance center is getting too much electrical information, as described above, some of it can "leak" over into the nausea center and stimulate it too.) The name for the vertigo that results from viral type infections is vestibular neuronitis, or labyrinthitis.

Another fairly common cause for vertigo that originates in the semi-circular canals is called otolithiasis, which roughly means "many rocks". This condition is caused by the formation of calcium deposits on the walls of the semi-circular canals over time (hence its association with advancing age) that can actually break loose from the walls of these canals and fall into the fluid along with the rock that is already there. These calcium deposits also act like rocks that, as a person moves, also stimulate the nerve endings in the canals. This results in conflicting sensory information being sent to the brain from the right versus the left set of semi-circular canals which produces the phenomenon of vertigo.

Other causes of vertigo that originate in the semi-circular canals are relatively rare. Meniere's disease, for example, affects hearing, causes pain in the ear, and is associated with both vertigo and a "roaring" sensation in the ear.

The only other source of vertigo, as stated earlier, is from malfunctions in the bundle of nerves that pass through the brainstem, electrically connecting the semi-circular canals with the higher processing area of the brain, the cortex. Malfunctions in this area are responsible for the remaining 10% of attacks of vertigo and are usually more serious because they are most often caused by strokes, tumors, and aneurysms located in the brainstem. Fortunately, vertigo that results from problems in the brainstem is much less common than the more benign vertigo that originates in the semi-circular canals.

It is not very difficult to tell whether vertigo is originating in the semi-circular canals or in the brainstem. Magnetic resonance imaging (MRI) is a test that produces images of the brainstem that will show if a person has had a stroke, or has a tumor or some other mass pushing on the brainstem. If this test is normal, as it usually is when a person has isolated vertigo without other symptoms, he or she can feel confident that the cause for the vertigo is located in the semi-circular canals and is benign. There is another test for diagnosing malfunctions in the brainstem called a brainstem auditory evoked response (BAER) test that is often used as a screening test for causes of vertigo, as it is much cheaper than an MRI, but it is not as reliable.

The easiest, and definitely the cheapest, way of diagnosing the origin of vertigo is to monitor the symptoms over a period of time. If the vertigo is intermittent with complete clearing of the symptoms in between spells of vertigo, or if the spells only occur when the head is moved from one position to another, then there is almost no chance that the vertigo originated in the brainstem but, rather, in the semi-circular canals instead. If the vertigo is the result of a stroke or tumor in the brainstem, for example, then one would expect the symptoms to be present all the time.

A person's response to medication for vertigo can also help predict in which of the two areas the vertigo originated. Meclizine is the medication ordinarily used to give resolution of the symptoms of vertigo. If meclizine relieves the symptoms of vertigo, then chances are that the vertigo was caused by a malfunction in the semi-circular canals. There is usually not much response to meclizine if the source of the vertigo is in the brainstem. There are anecdotal reports of various other medications that are purported to work to relieve the symptoms of vertigo, but none of them has withstood the test of time. There are other medications used to relieve the nausea that is sometimes associated with spells of vertigo, but these do nothing for the spinning sensation of vertigo.

Vertigo that results from otolithiasis, or "extra rocks" in the semi-circular canals, can sometimes be treated by tilting a person's head to one side and then leaning him or her backwards over a table at a specific angle. This maneuver is for the purpose of getting the extra rocks in the canals to float to the bottom of the semi-circular canals where they can then be eliminated more quickly. They usually will eventually find their way out of the semi-circular canals anyway, but this maneuver sometimes helps to speed up the process.

The most common presentation of vertigo is of a singular episode that occurs when a person leans over to pick up an object. It usually lasts for from a few seconds to a few minutes or so, and then resolves completely. This type presentation does not require any medical intervention. It is only when the spells continue to recur every few minutes or don't resolve after an hour or longer that they should be evaluated by a neurologist.

One might wonder why a malfunction, such as a stroke, in the higher brain processing area for balance does-n't cause vertigo. This is because there are two areas in the cortex of the brain that receive the information being sent from the semi-circular canals, one on the left side and one on the right side. If one side fails because of a stroke or other malfunction, the opposite side can still process the incoming sensory information from the semi-circular canals by way of the brainstem bundles of wires such that, ultimately, the information gets processed correctly. This can be thought of as a "back-up" system. If, however, both halves of the cortex of the brain that process balance infor-mation were affected by some malfunction, then the person would most likely have vertigo as a symptom. Of course, if a person had a malfunction that affected both halves of the cortex of the brain, vertigo would be the least of his or her worries.

LIGHTHEADEDNESS

Dizziness that occurs because of lightheadedness is usually related to a malfunction in some other part of the body that then exerts its effect on the brain by depriving the brain of an adequate blood supply. The only malfunc-tion that originates in the nervous system that causes light-headedness is an "autonomic" dysfunction.

The autonomic part of the nervous system is respon-sible for all the functions that we take for granted, such as controlling our heart rate, moving food through the diges-tive system, shivering when we are cold, and, for the pur-poses of this discussion, controlling the diameter of the blood vessels so that adequate supplies of blood are deliv-ered to various organs, such as the brain. Normally, when we stand up, the autonomic system causes the blood ves-sels in the neck and chest to constrict somewhat to provide more pressure on the blood in these vessels such that it can make it all the way to the brain instead of pooling in the lower half of the body from the effects of gravity. Shy-Draeger syndrome is the name of a neurologic disease that affects the ability of the autonomic nervous system to perform this task on the blood vessels. The result of this disease, as predicted, is a lightheaded feeling every time a person with Shy-Draeger syndrome goes from a lying or sitting position to a standing position.

A vaso-vagal response is a sudden dilation of the blood vessels in the neck or chest that then results in a sudden decrease in the blood pressure and subsequent blood flow to the brain. It can be caused by a frightening experience, (the autonomic part of the nervous system is responsible for our bodily responses to sudden emotional experiences) or may be caused by a sudden, intense pain, or a variety of other sudden emotional stressors that overstimulate the autonomic centers in the brain by sending an excessive amount of electrical current from the wires in the emotional areas of the brain to the autonomic areas, resulting in an exaggerated response by the autonomic system. Whatever the cause, the result of a vaso-vagal response is a feeling of lightheadedness at the least, and, if severe enough, can actually result in sudden loss of consciousness from the decreased blood flow to the brain.

There are other causes for a person's inability to control the diameter of the blood vessels going to the brain, resulting in lightheadedness, but these are not due to causes originating in the nervous system. For instance, people who have diabetes seem to be prone to having poor regulation of the diameter of blood vessels, and consequently, are frequently plagued by lightheadedness, especially in the later stages of this disease.

Occasionally, after emptying one's bladder, lightheadedness can result, especially in males, who usually stand during this function. As the bladder empties, a void is created inside the abdominal area. This decreases some of the pressure on the blood vessels in the abdominal cavity, resulting in a sudden reflex dilation of those blood vessels and a shunting of blood from the other areas of the body, especially from those areas above the heart (such as the brain) to the areas around the bladder. The net result of this action is a decrease in the amount of blood arriving at the brain, which results in lightheadedness.

One of the most common causes of lightheadedness is a malfunction within the heart that results in less than adequate pumping of blood out of this organ. Palpitations, or arrhythmias, result when the heart doesn't beat properly. Because of this, the blood is not forced out of the heart in a smooth, rhythmic pattern, but rather, it sloshes around within the heart. The result of this is less blood being pumped, which results in decreased bloodflow to the brain. With minor arrhythmias, lightheadedness is the result. With more profound arrhythmias, a person may actually lose consciousness, which will be discussed further in the next chapter.

You may wonder why, in some cases, a lack of adequate blood supply to the brain may cause confusion, as stated in a previous chapter, while in other cases, a lack of adequate blood supply to the brain may cause lightheadedness. The answer to this is a matter of degree. In order for confusion to result from a decreased blood flow to the brain, the condition has to be more severe. That is, the minimal decrease in the bloodflow to cause lightheadedness is not enough to cause confusion. Also, for confusion to result, the decrease in the bloodflow usually must persist for a longer period of time.

It may be starting to become clear that the causes for many of the various symptoms that are related to malfunctions in the nervous system are not all that different from one another, in spite of the sometimes vastly different ways the symptoms present themselves. As we move on to the following chapters, you will see that this phenomenon will tend to continue.

Chapter 4

Chapter 5
BLACKOUTS

A "blackout" refers to a brief loss of consciousness that is sudden in onset. The important words in this definition are "brief" and "sudden". A person who remains unconscious for an extended period of time would be more likely to have lapsed into coma rather than to have "blacked out". Also, a person who slowly drifts into the unconscious state would not ordinarily be described as having "blacked out", but rather, as having lapsed into coma as well.

Blackouts are not as uncommon as one might think. In a month's time, I may see as many as 10 or 15 patients with this complaint. Of course, the description of the blackout, as given by the patient, may not always be consistent with an actual loss of consciousness when he or she is questioned in depth about it. Probably the most common misconception that patients may have about blackouts occurs when they have severe vascular headaches that require them to lie down in a dark room for relief. If they fall asleep in the dark room, as they frequently will do with a vascular headache, they occasionally consider this to be a blackout from the headache, even though it is not.

When a person loses consciousness, either suddenly as with a blackout, or gradually, as in coma, this phenomenon is the result of abnormalities that occur within specific areas of the brain. If normal processing of electrical information by either the right or the left side of a part of the brainstem called the reticular activating system is interrupted, or if both halves of the higher brain (cortex) are interrupted at the same time, a loss of consciousness results. There is no other part of the brain or body that, if it malfunctions, will directly cause a loss of consciousness. Loss of consciousness can be caused by various other malfunctions, such as a heart arrhythmia where a less than adequate supply of blood is delivered to the brain, but these are all "indirect" causes of loss of consciousness because they exert their effects on the above areas of the brain related to maintaining the conscious state, rather than because they can cause unconsciousness without any effect on these areas of the brain. In other words, if a person is unconscious, there is 100% certainty that a malfunction has occurred in one or both halves of the brainstem where the reticular activating system is located, or in both halves of the cortex, either directly from a problem within these areas, or indirectly from a problem in another part of the body that ultimately affects the normal functioning of these specific areas of the brain.

The reticular activating system is located in a relatively small area in about the center of the brainstem. It is this area that generates the continuous pulses of current that can be channeled to the wires that activate the memory branches in our remote (permanent) memories, if you will recall the chapter dealing with memory. It would seem to make sense, then, that if something affects the ability of the reticular activating system to generate the current to keep the brain "active", then a loss of consciousness would result. A loss of consciousness may be a matter of degree of decreased activity in the reticular activating system. That is, with less and less activity in this area, a person may fall deeper and deeper into a state of unconsciousness until finally, the current is shut down completely. For example, when we are asleep, we are not consciously aware of our surroundings, but it is known that the reticular activating system is still generating currents in the various wires of the brain, although at a reduced rate. (This is why we have dreams. The current generator sends current over the wires at random without any specific direction, and the result is stimulation of various memory branches at random which we sometimes are able to reproduce when we awaken as a recollection of these "dreams". The randomness of the stimulation of memory branches is also why, when we are able to reproduce these patterns of memory stimulation when we are awake, they often don't make a lot of sense.) Sleep can therefore be thought of as a "mild" interruption in the ability of the brainstem's reticular activating system to generate electrical current. (There will be more about this in the chapter on sleep problems.) A blackout is a more severe interruption in the ability of the reticular activating system to generate current.

As stated above, there is one other area of the brain besides the reticular activating system of the brainstem that can cause a loss of consciousness if it malfunctions. This is the higher brain, or cortex. In this case, however, both halves of the cortex must be involved for an actual loss of consciousness to occur. (The importance of the involvement of both halves of the cortex will be seen later in this chapter when we discuss "strokes" as a cause of blackouts.) If the current generator is working fine, but the cortex is not, then the current that is being generated is not finding its way to areas of the brain where "awareness" of ourselves and our surroundings is located. This area of "awareness" is the cortex of the brain.

One might argue that a person who has severe

dementia, such as Alzheimer's disease, is not aware of himself or herself, nor of his or her surroundings, but is not considered to be unconscious. In this case, although the person is not aware, he or she is still able to "react" to stimuli. For instance, if one waves a hand in front of a demented person's face, he or she will blink. Unconsciousness, if caused by a malfunction in both halves of the cortex, involves essentially all of the cortex, including the parts used for moving muscles, not just certain parts, such as the memory areas, the sensory areas, or the motor areas that are involved with movements.

CAUSES OF BLACKOUTS

Although, as mentioned above, blackouts are not all that uncommon, the causes for them are relatively few. First we will discuss the most common causes of blackouts, then the less common causes, and finally, the misconceptions about diseases that are thought to cause blackouts, but that actually do not.

When I am asked to see a patient because of blackout spells, nearly 100% of the time the cause is from one of three phenomena. In children and in younger adults, the most common cause is seizures. In older patients, the most common cause is episodic periods of decreased blood flow to the brain, either from autonomic dysfunction, in which the blood vessels carrying blood to the brain do not constrict as they are supposed to, such as when a person stands up, for example, or from the third most common cause, heart arrhythmias, which cause turbulence within the heart leading to less blood being pumped out of the heart and to the brain. The workup of the person with blackouts, then, involves looking for seizure activity, looking for abnormalities in the autonomic nervous system, and looking for abnormalities in the heart.

Seizures occur when there is an excess of electrical

activity in the brain, rather than a shortage of activity. So far in this discussion, we have been concerned with losses of consciousness resulting from too little activity occurring in the two areas of the brain that are concerned with keeping us alert. When a seizure occurs, electrical activity spreads to essentially all the wires located in a particular area of the brain, such that the normal function of that particular area is abolished because the area of the brain involved in the excess of electrical activity can not interact with incoming electrical information from wires outside that area. Remember, everything we think and do is related to the interaction of the various communication and memory wires in the brain, and when a specific area of the brain can no longer communicate with other areas of the brain, either because of a lack or an excess of electrical current, it is effectively "removed", either temporarily, or permanently, from the nervous system. When a seizure remains localized to a small, specific area of the brain, the patient may exhibit various signs, such as twitching of a corner of the mouth if the part of the brain that controls mouth movements is involved, or "rage" type responses if the emotional areas of the brain are involved, for example. The excess of electrical activity that occurs in the wires of the brain when a seizure occurs is able to be transmitted away from the involved area of the brain to other parts of the brain, or to various muscle groups. It is only incoming electrical information that is stopped because of the seizure activity in the involved area of the brain. If a seizure spreads to involve more and more of the brain, eventually, there will be enough of the brain involved such that unconsciousness will result. This is because with more and more involvement of the brain, less and less incoming electrical information is able to be processed, and as stated earlier, with inability of the brain to process incoming electrical information, unconsciousness results. (Remember that the area of the brain involved with the seizure activity can send information but can't receive information.)

A seizure may spread rapidly from its area of origin to the rest of the brain, in which case consciousness is lost immediately, or may spread slowly to the rest of the brain, such that the patient may exhibit signs that indicate that a seizure is beginning sometime before he or she actually loses consciousness. In some cases, a person may lose consciousness from a seizure without actually exhibiting the jerking type movements usually associated with the excess electrical current that finds its way away from the area of the brain involved with the seizure down through the brainstem, then the spinal cord, and then out the peripheral nerves to the muscles. In these cases, it is not as obvious to a witness that the person is actually having a seizure, which makes the diagnosis for the cause of the blackout more difficult.

Although a first seizure is a frightening experience, both to the person who has it, and to a person who observes it, the causes of seizures are usually not serious. By far, the two most common causes of seizures in adults are metabolic abnormalities, such as too little magnesium or calcium in the blood, and from the side effects of medications. Most people are afraid that if they have a first seizure as an adult, they must have a tumor in their brains. This is actually a very rare cause of seizures in both adults and children.

A CAT scan, which is an X-ray of the brain, and an electroencephalogram (EEG), which shows if abnormal electrical activity is occurring in the brain, are usually performed on patients that have had a seizure, or in patients who are suspected of having had a seizure, to determine if any obvious abnormalities exist in the brain that might have triggered the blackout. In my experience, more than 80% of these two tests are normal, even in patients who have had an obvious seizure as a cause for their losses of consciousness. This of course doesn't mean that the blackout never occurred, but rather that the cause is probably not serious. For instance, in children, most seizures probably occur because of a "short" in one of the millions of wires in the brain, which then spreads to the surrounding wires eventually causing a seizure. The brain is not completely formed until a child is 7 or 8 years old, and during the time prior to this, when various connections are being formed by the wires that make up the brain, some "bad" connections may be made that result in a tendency for the child to have seizures until the situation spontaneously corrects itself. When one thinks about all the millions of connections that are made between the various wires of the brain as the brain is forming, it would seem that a logical question might ask why there aren't more people with seizures.

Autonomic dysfunction was first mentioned in the last chapter when discussing causes of lightheadedness. It refers to the part of the nervous system that contains the wires that are used for keeping our bodies running properly. It is responsible for keeping our hearts beating, for moving the food through our intestines, for causing us to shiver when we are cold to help heat our bodies up, for sweating to cool our bodies off, for emotional responses, and, in the case of this discussion, for dilating and constricting blood vessels in order to regulate the flow of blood through them.

The term "autonomic", which sounds like "automatic", refers to just this very concept. That is, the autonomic nervous system works automatically without any voluntary efforts on our part. When it goes awry, we also cannot consciously correct it. This is the case when, for instance, we hear some news that is emotionally upsetting. This causes an increase in activity in the autonomic nervous system, which is involved in emotions, and some of this electrical activity "leaks" to the blood vessels where it causes them to dilate. The blood then drains from the brain if the person is in an upright position, and he or she blacks out.

In most cases where a person blacks out without any prior "upsetting" news, and has no previous history of seizures nor heart arrhythmias, autonomic malfunction is the cause. There is a test available in which a person is strapped to a table that rotates from a flat to standing position while he or she is observed. In cases of autonomic malfunction, the patient's blood pressure does not respond appropriately when the person is turned to the upright position, and he or she is actually seen to black out on the table. This verifies the cause as a malfunction in the autonomic nervous system. Medications, such as propranolol and trazadone, which can affect the current in the wires of the autonomic nervous system, can sometimes help remedy this situation. In some cases where medications don't seem to help, the person with an autonomic nervous system malfunction is simply told to get up slowly from lying to sitting position, or from sitting to standing position. This usually helps at least somewhat to relieve the symptoms.

As explained in the previous chapter, an autonomic malfunction can cause lightheadedness if it is a mild malfunction, but if it is more severe, an actual blackout may occur. Many of the symptoms discussed in this book, although different in their presentations, are only really different in the degree of their effects on the wires that carry electrical current from one place to another in the nervous system.

The third most common cause of blackouts, heart arrhythmias, has also been mentioned in the previous chapter as a cause of lightheadedness. As with autonomic malfunction, the degree of heart arrhythmias predicts whether the patient will black out or will only become lightheaded.

To determine if a person is having arrhythmias, a holter monitor is used. This is a device that keeps track of every heartbeat for 24 hours in a small cassette, which can then be played back by a heart specialist to look for any evidence of abnormal heartbeats during those 24 hours. The device is portable and is worn on a belt. Of course, if the person doesn't have any abnormal heartbeats during the time that the device is worn, it will register as a normal study. Usually, however, a person is able to relate that he or she was having unusual type heart beats prior to blacking out if this is the underlying cause.

Trauma may cause a blackout. This cause is usually fairly obvious because of lacerations or bumps on the head, and needs no further attention in this discussion except to point out that the reason a person loses consciousness with a head injury that does not cause any visible damage to the brain itself is because as the brain gets "thrown around" inside the skull, the chemicals that cause the current in the wires to flow from one wire to the next get mixed up such that they are not at the proper concentrations to keep the current flowing in the wires in a normal way. If the current doesn't flow properly in the reticular activating system in the brainstem, or in both halves of the cortex of the brain, then a blackout results.

When a larger blood vessel suddenly breaks open in the brain, such as when an aneurysm ruptures, (an aneurysm is a bubble that forms on a blood vessel where the wall of that blood vessel has weakened) a person may suddenly black out. However, if a person blacks out from a broken blood vessel in the brain, he or she will not wake up after a few minutes as expected with a blackout. The person will become comatose. Almost always, a ruptured blood vessel in the brain will give a warning sign that this has occurred before the person loses consciousness. This warning sign is a severe headache that is usually worse than any headache the person has ever experienced. This cause for loss of consciousness is almost never confused with the three most common causes mentioned earlier.

A very common misconception is that strokes frequently cause blackouts. Almost 90% of strokes are caused by blockages in the blood vessels that carry blood from the heart to the wires that make up the brain. The other 10% of strokes are caused by broken blood vessels that allow the blood to leak out into the brain. For the most common type of stroke to cause a blackout, the blood vessels that go to the reticular activating system of the brainstem would have to be involved with the blockage. This is very unlikely because of the arrangement of the blood supply in that area of the brain. Also, strokes almost never affect more than one blood vessel in the brain at a time, and if one occurs because of a blockage in the cortex of the brain, which is the only other area that can produce loss of consciousness if the electric current is interrupted, it would not affect both halves of the cortex at the same time. There are no blood vessels that go to both halves of the cortex. As you may remember, for a loss of consciousness to occur from a malfunction in the cortex, both halves must be involved at the same time. If, on the other hand, a person has one of the rarer types of strokes that involve a broken blood vessel that leaks blood into the brain in large enough quantities such that the brainstem or cortex becomes compressed to the point that consciousness is lost, this would not be consistent with a blackout because this would not be a brief loss of consciousness. It would be more consistent with lapsing into coma. If a person has a blackout with return to wakefulness after a brief period of time, this blackout is simply not caused by a stroke.

In summation, blackouts are brief, sudden losses of consciousness that are almost always caused by either seizures (especially in children), autonomic nervous system malfunctions, or from heart arrhythmias, the latter two causes especially seen in older individuals.

Chapter 6
NUMBNESS AND TINGLING

Second to headaches, the most common neurologic complaint seems to be numbness or tingling, which may be confined to one extremity, two or more extremities, both arms or both legs, both feet or hands, the face, or all over. The characteristics of the numbness or tingling feeling are not nearly as important for purposes of diagnosing the cause of the symptoms as the location of the numbness or tingling sensation.

Unlike most of the symptoms in the preceding chapters, numbness and tingling can not be localized to one or two isolated areas of the nervous system. A person can experience numbness or tingling because of a malfunction in the brain, including the higher brain (cortex) and the lower brain (brainstem), the spinal cord, or the peripheral wires themselves. Numbness and tingling are sensory symptoms, however, and so the only parts of the nervous system that can be involved with these symptoms would necessarily be the parts that deal with sensory information. These would be the wires in which a current is begun by light touch, pain, heat, cold, pressure, and vibration in the mechanoreceptors located in the very ends of the wires. Remember, these are called mechanoreceptors because the current is begun at the very ends of these sensory wires by mechanically manipulating the tip of the nerve by one of the methods mentioned above. For instance, if a sensory wire that transports pain information to the brain is mechanically manipulated at its tip by a knife, the knife starts the current flowing as it interacts with the receptor at the tip of the wire by either bending the receptor, cutting it, or stretching it. If the same knife interacts with a pressure receptor, the electrical current that is started flowing towards the brain travels up a pressure sensing wire, and when the current arrives at the brain, it is perceived as pressure rather than pain. Pressure receptors are much easier to stimulate than pain receptors, which is why a person would only feel pressure sensation with a light push on the skin with a knife and pain sensation with a heavier push on the skin. Pain sensation is also given top priority for processing in the brain over any of the other sensory modalities. This is because if a pain wire is stimulated, this means that there is damage being done to the body and something needs to be done immediately to correct the situation. Returning to the example of the knife, once the pain wires are stimulated by the pushing of the knife on the skin, a person is no longer as aware of the pressure sensation from the knife because the pain sensation takes priority by tying up the wires in the brain and brainstem with processing the incoming pain information.

As sensory information passes from the tip of the peripheral wires located everywhere throughout the body up the peripheral wires to the spinal cord, then to the brainstem, and finally to the cortex of the brain, a malfunction in any of these four areas can produce the sensation of numbness or tingling. It may sound nearly impossible to locate the exact area where the malfunction has occurred, but, as stated at the beginning of this chapter, the location of the numbness or tingling sensation gives the best clue as to its area of origin.

We will divide the four areas into two sections, the central nervous system, which includes the cortex of the brain, the brainstem, and the spinal cord, and the peripheral nervous system, which includes all the wires after they leave the spinal cord. The division is made in this manner because it is usually easier to differentiate whether symptoms of numbness and tingling originated in the central nervous system or the peripheral nervous system. This, then, can potentially save the patient a lot of money by avoiding unnecessary tests on the wrong system. First we will discuss the presentation and causes of numbness and tingling that arise from malfunctions in the central nervous system, and then we will discuss the possible malfunctions that lead to numbness and tingling arising in the peripheral nervous system.

CENTRAL NERVOUS SYSTEM

Numbness or tingling that arises because of a malfunction in the central nervous system is essentially always confined to either the right or left side, but not both. If someone complains of both arms or both legs tingling, we can usually be sure that the primary problem is not located in the cortex of the brain, the brainstem, or spinal cord. (It should be mentioned that there are some hereditary diseases that can cause degeneration of the sensory processing areas of both halves of the brain and spinal cord, resulting in both arms or both legs being involved, but these are not only very rare, they also are almost always associated with other symptoms that make them easier to diagnose as originating in the central nervous system. In my practice, I may see one or two of these cases in a span of three or four years, which attests to their rarity. I have never seen one in which numbness or tingling was the only symptom.)

The most common cause of numbness or tingling arising from the central nervous system is stroke. This type of numbness is not associated with any pain, comes about suddenly, and is more diffuse in nature, affecting an entire arm or leg, for example, rather than isolated parts of the arm or leg, such as certain fingers or certain toes. One might wonder why the brain can't effect isolated movements or sensations in all the various parts of the body. In actuality, the brain can effect isolated movements and sensations, but because of the architectural arrangement of the blood supply to the brain, when a stroke occurs, it is essentially impossible for the stroke to affect such a small area in the sensory part of the brain such that only an individual part of a leg or arm, for example, is affected. In experiments done several years ago by neurosurgeons while operating on the brain of a patient in the awake state, individual wires of the cortex of the brain were stimulated directly with an electric current from a very thin wire, and in this way, tiny areas of various parts of the body could be made to "feel" a numb or tingling sensation.

Seizures can also cause isolated symptoms of numbness and tingling, if they happen to occur in the sensory area of the cortex of the brain without spreading to any other parts of the brain. Unlike a stroke, which causes the sensation of numbness and tingling because the sensory information from the peripheral wires cannot reach the cortex of the brain, its final destination after traveling from the peripheral mechanoreceptor where it started, a seizure causes a feeling of numbness and tingling because of overstimulation of the sensory area of the cortex of the brain. It may seem paradoxical that the same symptoms can be caused not only by an inability of the cortex of the brain to be stimulated electrically, but also by overstimulation of the same area. However, when one remembers that everything we consciously perceive (sense) is through the electrical activity that travels throughout the cortex of the brain, it becomes easier to understand. That is, in the case of damage to the cortex of the brain, peripheral current never arrives at an area where it can be perceived, resulting in the numbness, or "lack" of feeling. When a seizure occurs, however, one feels a tingling sensation because of stimulation of the sensory cortex directly without actually starting the current flow from the usual starting point, the mechanoreceptor in the peripheral wire. When a seizure occurs, the whole system is bypassed by stimulating the cortex of the brain directly such that there is a perception that a peripheral receptor was stimulated, even though it was not. In other words, with seizures, what the cortex of the brain "feels" is not really occurring in the peripheral areas, while with strokes, what the cortex of the brain is not "feeling" really is being felt in the peripheral areas, the result of which, in both cases, is ultimately an abnormal feeling of numbness or tingling.

Other causes of numbness and tingling that occur in the brain or brainstem would include tumors and other space occupying masses. In these cases, the numbness and tingling are slow in onset, rather than of sudden onset, such as with a stroke. If a person relates a history of slow, gradual onset of worsening numbness or tingling over a period of several weeks or months that is confined to one side of the body and is not associated with pain in the affected area, then a tumor in the brain is a possible cause of the symptoms.

It should be mentioned that although "pain" is perceived and evaluated in the cortex of the brain, it cannot be elicited by directly stimulating the cortex of the brain. This is because what is finally perceived as pain in the cortex of the brain is the result of the interaction of other wires within the brain with the current that originally traveled up a pain wire towards the brain. That is, the "pain" that is finally perceived by the cortex is the result of several modifications of the incoming electrical pain signal such that it can travel to many areas rather than traveling along specific wires to a specific part of the cortex of the brain where pain perception would be located, as with all the other sensory modalities. In some people, an incoming pain signal may be amplified so that a seemingly minor cause for pain elicits a very strong reaction to this pain signal, while in others, a large quantity of incoming pain current from the peripheral nerves, as from a broken leg, may be modified in the cortex so that the final perception of the pain is of a minor nature. We can actually "learn" to modify pain signals so that the pain we perceive is more or less intense than in another person with the same type injury. The result of all this is that ultimately, the pain that is finally perceived is the result of the interaction of several wires within the brain, and therefore cannot be elicited by stimulating, or damaging, a specific wire in the cortex of the brain where pain signals may be processed. In other words, unlike all other sensory information, there is no one specific area in the cortex of the brain where pain signals are received. The perception of pain by each of us is the result of the interaction of various wires within the cortex of the brain with a pain signal from one of the peripheral wires when it reaches the brain.

The important part of this discussion about pain, for purposes of this chapter, is that if a person experiences pain along with numbness or tingling, the origin of the numbness or tingling is not in the brain because the brain cannot initiate pain signals, either in the normal state, or in the diseased state.

It seems that there are always exceptions to every rule, however, and in this case, there is also an exception which is very rare. A malfunction in a very isolated part of the brainstem can cause severe pain symptoms that may or may not be associated with numbness or tingling. Usually, though, there are either many other symptoms also associated with the intense pain, or the pain is the only symptom.

I have never seen a case where a malfunction in this area caused only pain along with numbness or tingling. There are no exceptions to this rule in the cortex of the brain, however.

Other than strokes, seizures, and space occupying masses, such as tumors, hemorrhages, and cysts, there are no other important causes of numbness and tingling that originate in the central nervous system. If one suspects that symptoms of numbness or tingling are arising in the central nervous system, an MRI will almost always diagnose the cause. In the case of seizures as a cause, an EEG will often make the diagnosis.

PERIPHERAL NERVOUS SYSTEM

There are many and varied causes for numbness and tingling that occur because of malfunctions in the peripheral nervous system. They can occur on both sides of the body at the same time, or may occur on one side or one extremity at a time. First, we will discuss the causes of numbness and tingling that occur on both sides of the body at one time, and then we will discuss the causes of numbness and tingling that occur on one side or in one extremity at a time.

For all practical purposes, any numbness or tingling that occurs on both sides of the body at the same time has its ultimate origin in the circulatory system, which supplies nutrients to the nerves by way of the constant blood flow to all the various areas of the body. When a feeling of numbness or tingling occurs on both sides, it almost always occurs in the same areas on the opposite sides, such as in both feet or both hands. This is because the circulations on the two sides of the body are nearly mirror images of each other, and if one foot, for example, is deprived of blood because of a weak heart, chances are that the other foot will suffer the same fate because of its similar blood vessel distribution and distance from the heart.

When any part of the body does not receive the proper amount of nutrients from a less than adequate supply of them by way of the blood, the sensory nerves in that area are the first to feel the effects of this problem, which makes sense, since the sensory nerves are what let the brain know what is going on with the rest of the body at any given time. The brain then acts upon this information in whatever way is appropriate. For instance, if a person is out in the cold without enough protective covering for the feet, the blood vessels in the feet begin to constrict to keep the blood from flowing through these cold areas so that the temperature of the blood in the body doesn't ultimately become reduced from heat loss through the feet. When the blood flow to the feet is reduced, the sensory wires in the feet are deprived of the nutrients from the blood and they are then prevented from sending normal sensory signals to the brain which results in a feeling of numbness in the nutrient deprived area. It is interesting to note that while all the usual sensory wires have decreased flow of electrical information, or current, to the brain when deprived of nutrients, the sensory wires that send pain signals become more active in sending signals at first when they are affected by adverse conditions. This is a protective mechanism in that as these increased pain signals arrive at the brain for processing, they are very motivating for getting us to do something (warming the feet) to eliminate the pain signals from continuing. Of course, if nothing is done and the process of depriving the feet of an adequate blood supply continues, even the pain signals will eventually be prevented from continuing due to the lack of energy supply.

As mentioned above, a malfunctioning heart can cause numbness and tingling on both sides of the body, and usually in the same areas of the two sides that are affected. The symptoms are usually noticed in the areas that are the farthest away from the heart, as this is where the blood pressure would necessarily be the lowest. The lower the blood pressure, the less blood (and nutrients) there is being delivered to that area. If someone has a complaint of numbness or tingling in both feet or both hands, a heart problem is one of the first causes that is usually considered.

Diabetes may be an even more frequent cause of numbness and tingling that occurs on both sides of the body at the same time. Although diabetes is a disease that affects the body's ability to handle sugar properly, it exerts its bad effects on the body by altering the blood carrying capacity of the blood vessels, and therefore, can affect any part of the body, since every part of the body relies on the blood continuously for nutrients. As with heart problems causing a compromised blood delivery system, diabetes also causes the blood vessels with the poorest blood supply to become affected first. These are usually the ones that are the farthest away from the heart, such as in the feet and hands.

Medications can cause numbness and tingling and this is usually seen on both sides of the body at the same time. Chemotherapy medications used for treating cancer are notorious for causing numbness and tingling because of their toxic effects on the peripheral nerves.

Usually, if a medication is the cause of numbness and tingling, it is a medication that has been recently started, rather than one that a person has been taking for years. In fact, when I see a patient who has a complaint of numbness or tingling that is of recent onset and is about the same on both sides of the body, and if they have also been started on a new medication within the previous few weeks, I first either discontinue that particular medication, or change it to an alternate one before doing any further neurologic testing. Most of the time, this corrects the problem.

One of the most common causes of numbness and tingling that affects both sides of the body, and is usually seen in the more peripheral areas, such as in the hands and feet, is atherosclerosis. This is a disease of the blood vessels, usually the result of chronic high blood pressure or chronically elevated cholesterol, in which the blood vessels become corroded and thickened with hard, rock-like deposits that prevent the proper amount of blood from traveling through the affected blood vessels. As with heart problems and diabetes, the blood vessels located the farthest distance from the heart where the pressure on the blood is the lowest, and also the smallest blood vessels, which don't have a lot of room within them in the first place to allow a buildup of abnormal deposits, are the most affected by atherosclerosis. The result of the decreased flow of blood in these areas is a lack of nutrients delivered to the wires in the same areas which results in their inability to transmit electrical impulses appropriately to the brain for further processing, and a feeling of numbness or tingling results.

Numbness or tingling that results from abnormalities in the blood vessels, such as from atherosclerosis, diabetes, and chronic high blood pressure are not treatable once they have occurred.

Numbness and tingling that occurs on one side of the body and has its origin in the peripheral nervous system is usually due to compression of the wire at some point between the spinal cord, where the peripheral wire originates, and the very end of the wire, usually in the skin somewhere.

The most common place where a wire may be compressed, or pinched, in the arm, is in the wrist, the elbow, or in the neck.

Carpal tunnel syndrome is the most common cause of symptoms of numbness or tingling that occurs in a hand only. It can occur because of chronic repetitive type movements of the hand and wrist or may be genetic in origin. The wrist is made up of several small bones and the wire that travels from the hand, then across the wrist, then up the arm, travels in a fairly precarious position as it crosses the wrist. It lies in a groove between the bones of the wrist where it is very prone to being pinched between these bones when there is a lot of twisting type activity done with the hand. Genetically, some people have a narrower groove through which this wire travels and are therefore more prone to having the wire become pinched with any strenuous type activity with that hand and wrist.

There is another wire that travels to the hand that passes over a bone in the elbow which makes it prone to being compressed by that bone in the elbow. When we hit our "funny bone", this is the wire that gets compressed between the bone in the elbow and the object that we bumped the elbow against. If the fourth and fifth fingers of one hand are numb or tingling, this wire is the one that is involved. However, if the thumb and first two fingers are involved with numbness and tingling, then the wire that causes carpal tunnel syndrome is the one that is involved.

A third area where a peripheral wire is prone to being compressed that causes numbness or tingling in an arm or hand is in the neck. The wire is in a vulnerable position as it exits from the spinal cord to begin along its pathway down the arm and can be compressed by three different tissues in this particular area. These are bone, cartilage, and muscle tissue, and a malfunction in any of these three tissues can result in compression of the wire in the neck. (This will be covered in detail in the chapter on neck and back pain.)

The most common place where a wire may be compressed, or pinched, in the leg is in the outer part of the knee or in the low back area. As in the arm, there is a wire that passes between two bones on the outside of the knee in a very small groove. When someone is injured on the outside of the knee, or in some cases, when a person lies on his or her side for too long a period of time, the most common cause of which is the result of passing out from overindulgence in alcohol, this wire is compressed between two bones in the knee and results in numbness or tingling in the foot or lower leg, if mild, or an actual weakness if more severe. (Remember, it takes more pressure on a peripheral wire to cause weakness than to cause numbness and tingling because the wires travel in bundles and the sensory wires are located around the outside of the bundle and are compressed first by outside pressure, while the wires that move the muscles are located on the inside of the bundles of wires and are therefore more protected from being compressed.)

Wires can also be compressed in the low back in the same manner as in the neck. That is, the bone, muscle, and cartilage that are in close proximity to the wires as they exit from the spinal cord can compress the wires when these three tissues malfunction.

The treatment for compression of the wires at the elbow, wrist, and outside part of the knee involve relatively minor surgical procedures. In each case, the wire is moved out of the area where it is being compressed to another less confining position. People do remarkably well with these surgical corrections. The treatment for compression of the wires as they exit from the spinal cord depends on whether it is bone, muscle, or cartilage that is pinching the wire. As stated above, this will be covered in the chapter on back and neck pain.

There is another cause for numbness and tingling that typically causes these symptoms in one or both hands (usually both) and in the face, usually the area around the mouth. It is unusual in that it involves both the central and peripheral nervous systems and is the result of an anxiety or stress related syndrome. In these cases, a person, because of an anxious or stressful situation, has a tendency to breathe one or two times more per minute than the usual 13 or 14 breaths per minute. This is called hyperventilation, but is not what we ordinarily think of as "hyperventilating", as it is nearly impossible to tell that the person is even taking any more breaths than usual. The person's body, on the other hand, is very aware of these extra breaths, and tries to do something about the excess oxygen that is being delivered from the lungs into the bloodstream from these extra breaths which, over a period of time, add up to a lot of extra oxygen in the body. Too much oxygen reaching the tissues in the body is toxic and can cause damage. The way that the body prevents an excess of oxygen from reaching the tissues is to constrict the blood vessels so that not so much of the oxygen-rich blood reaches the tissues. Unfortunately, this also means that other nutrients in the blood are temporarily prevented from reaching the tissues too. The sensory wires of the face and hands are most sensitive to this closing down of the blood vessels and numbness and tingling in these areas is the result. Of course, if persons voluntarily hyperventilated as hard as they could, for as long as they could, the blood vessels would constrict so tightly from the large excess of oxygen that there wouldn't be enough blood reaching the brain and the person would pass out. The almost imperceptible one or two extra breaths per minute that occur with an anxiety produced hyperventilation only cause mild symptoms as described above.

The reason that the phenomenon of hyperventilation is produced by an anxiety type situation is because anxiety causes (or is caused by) excess electrical activity in the brain. This excess electrical current in the brain can find its way to any of the wires in the brain. If it travels to the emotional centers, a panic type situation may result. If it travels to the part of the brainstem that controls the rate of breathing, then extra breaths may be triggered by the brainstem as it sends more current down the wires that go to the diaphragm that moves the lungs in and out.

This phenomenon of subtle hyperventilation causing numbness and tingling in the hands and mouth that is triggered by anxiety is usually very easy to diagnose but is also one of the hardest diagnoses to convince a patient that he or she has. The patients have a tendency to assume that the physician is making "light" of their condition rather than finding out what is "really" wrong. Unfortunately, part of the anxiety situation usually entails a feeling of doom, or that things are out of control, and being told that this is the diagnosis seems to compound these feelings. Antidepressants are the usual agents used to control this problem, and they work quite well when the patient can be convinced of the diagnosis.

To summarize, numbness and tingling can usually be localized to a problem in the central nervous system if located on one side of the body and involving an entire limb, or in the peripheral nervous system if involving both sides of the body or isolated parts of an arm or leg. Problems with circulation are the most common causes of numbness and tingling that affect both sides of the body, while stroke is the most common cause of numbness and tingling that affects an entire side of the body.

Chapter 7
WEAKNESS

Weakness, like numbness and tingling, can arise from malfunctions in any part of the nervous system, including the brain, the spinal cord, and the peripheral wires. Unlike the sensory wires that carry information towards the brain from the peripheral areas, however, the wires involved with weakness carry information away from the brain towards the muscles. In this chapter, the causes for malfunctions in this specific class of wires will be discussed.

There is also another cause for weakness that has to be included along with malfunctions in the wires themselves, and this is malfunctions within the muscles that the wires stimulate to contract as the electrical impulses reach the muscles. In other words, diseases of the muscles themselves can also cause weakness.

By far the most common type of weakness that I see is of a generalized nature involving both arms and both legs and is of gradual onset, usually over a few weeks. It typically occurs in someone over the age of thirty. The cause for this weakness is about equally divided between medications that the person may be taking and depression.

I would estimate that approximately 90% of all patients who have a complaint of generalized weakness are found to have one of these two causes as the origin of the weakness.

The most common type of weakness that affects one side of the body, either one arm, one leg, one side of the face, or combinations of these three areas on the same side of the body, is stroke. In my experience, over 90% of one-sided symptoms of weakness fall under this diagnosis.

Another fairly common cause of weakness, which can be either generalized in origin or related to one side or one extremity, is pain. In this case, however, the person does not really have an actual "weakness", but rather, a phenomenon called "guarding", which is a protection from movement of a part of the body because of the pain associated with moving that body part. Arthritis is the overwhelming cause in most cases of weakness originating in this way.

The four causes of weakness mentioned above, medications, depression, stroke, and guarding because of pain associated with moving a body part, account for about 95% of all weakness that I am asked to evaluate in my practice. Usually, it is not too difficult to determine which of these four is the culprit. If only these four possibilities were used in making a diagnosis, 95% of the time it would be easy. Unfortunately, the other 5% of the time, the diagnosis can be much more difficult. In this chapter, we will discuss not only the above mentioned causes for weakness, but the other causes as well. As with the chapter on causes of numbness and tingling, we will divide the causes into central nervous system origin, peripheral nervous system origin, and a third category, malfunctions in the muscles themselves.

CENTRAL NERVOUS SYSTEM

As mentioned previously, the central nervous system consists of the wires that make up the higher centers of the brain, also called the "cortex" of the brain, the brainstem and its associated areas, such as the cerebellum (which altogether will be referred to as the "brainstem" for purposes of this discussion), and the spinal cord.

Impulses of electric current that are involved in moving muscles all begin in a relatively small area of the cortex of the brain. Every voluntary movement that we make originates in this narrow strip. It is located about in the center of each of the halves of the cortex and is about one half inch wide and 3 or 4 inches long in both halves of the brain. The strip on the left side of the brain initiates movements on the right side of the body and the strip on the right side of the brain initiates movements on the left side of the body. After an electric current is generated in one of the wires in this area, it next passes through the brainstem where it is modified by brainstem influences so that the ultimate movement is smooth and rhythmic rather than jerking in nature. From the brainstem, the electric impulse travels down the spinal cord and then out from the spinal cord by way of a peripheral wire until it reaches the target muscle, where the electric current causes the muscle to contract.

ACUTE WEAKNESS OF CENTRAL NERVOUS SYSTEM ORIGIN

As mentioned earlier, stroke is the most common cause of acute weakness that originates in the central nervous system (and affects only one side of the body). A stroke can occur either in the cortex of the brain along the strip of wires mentioned above that is involved in initiating impulses to ultimately move muscles, or in the brainstem, through which the impulses of electric current pass on the

101

way to the muscles. Strokes can also occur in the spinal cord, but these are extremely rare. Of the strokes that occur in the cortex of the brain and in the brainstem, about 90% of them are caused by blockages in the blood vessels that carry nutrients to the brain. These blockages can occur from occlusion of the interior of the blood vessels with cholesterol deposits that have accumulated over the years, or other "junk" that has accumulated within the interior of the blood vessel opening to the point where the blood is eventually prevented from flowing.

These blockages can also occur if a small blood clot that has formed in some other part of the circulation system breaks loose and travels along until it finally reaches a small enough blood vessel where it can become stuck, blocking the blood flow downstream from where it is stuck. This also results in a stroke if the clot gets stuck in one of the blood vessels in the brain.

The two most common areas from which these small blood clots become dislodged and start floating downstream to eventually cause a stroke are in the heart itself and in the main blood vessels in the neck that carry blood to the brain. In fact, when a person has a stroke, there will usually be tests performed to determine if there are any clots stuck to the inside walls of the heart or the inside walls of the blood vessels in the neck, and if so, they are usually removed, either by surgery or by using blood thinners for the purpose of dissolving them so that further strokes can be prevented. At the point when the blood actually stops flowing, a stroke will occur. This is why it is imperative to keep the blood vessels of the brain, as well as the blood vessels that feed into the blood vessels of the brain, open.

The remaining 10% of strokes are caused by a break in one of the blood vessels in the brain, usually due to too much pressure within the blood vessel in people who have a history of high blood pressure, or from straining at some task, which acutely raises the blood pressure to sometimes dangerous levels, or from ruptured aneurysms, which are small weak areas in the blood vessel walls that cause the blood vessels to be pushed out like small balloons in these areas.

When someone has a fairly sudden onset of weakness on one side of the body that is not associated with pain, the most likely cause of this one-sided weakness is stroke. (Remember that the brain cannot initiate pain sensation within itself since there is not one particular area of the brain where pain sensation is located but is rather the modification of incoming pain signals that the brain reacts with that gives one the sensation, or perception, of pain.)

Another possible cause for sudden onset of weakness that originates in the brain would include complicated migraine, which is the result of spasms of the blood vessels within the brain, sometimes so severe that the flow of blood is impeded enough that symptoms of weakness can result if the blood vessel that spasms is one that supplies the part of the brain that initiates, or is involved with, moving muscles. In the case of complicated migraine, the spasming of the blood vessel in the closed position is then followed by a spasming in the wide open position, which stretches the pain nerve endings in the blood vessels, and triggers the severe headache that is associated with complicated migraine. Sometimes, the only way to tell a complicated migraine from a stroke is by the headache that is associated with the complicated migraine that does not occur with the stroke. Also, the weakness that results with complicated migraine is not permanent, and usually lasts less than a day.

CHRONIC WEAKNESS OF CENTRAL NERVOUS SYSTEM ORIGIN

Chronic weakness that has its origin in the brain is

more diverse in its possible causes. Infections in the brain, tumors of the brain, multiple sclerosis, depression, blood vessel malformations, and genetic causes, especially in children, can all cause weakness, ultimately. Infections of the brain, if diffuse, such as meningitis or encephalitis, usually cause other symptoms along with a generalized weakness, including pain, stiff neck, and especially, a change in the person's level of consciousness. However, some infections, such as abscesses in the brain, parasite infections (various "worms" that are rare in this country), and fungal infections, such as those obtained by working in close contact with various birds, can be localized to specific small areas of the brain, including the areas associated with the movement of muscles. All of these infectious causes work similarly on the brain to cause the damage to the areas of the brain that move muscles. That is, the organisms involved in these infectious processes either destroy the brain cells or they cause an inflammatory reaction in that area of the brain that inhibits the proper delivery of nutrients to that area from the blood due to the swelling and congestion with white blood cells in that area. The white blood cells are there to try to fight off the infection, but unfortunately, the large numbers of them present can also cause congestion of the usual smooth workings of the nutrient delivery system of the blood resulting in weakness, if the part of the brain involved happens to be associated with movement of muscles. If the damage to the brain is not complete, the weakness may resolve once the infected state resolves. If the damage is more complete, the affected part of the brain may never return to its previous level of functioning and the person may be permanently weak. Of course, this can occur in any part of the brain, including the sensory areas, in which case, the person would have symptoms of numbness or tingling rather than weakness.

The treatment for infectious causes of weakness

would include antibiotics to kill the offending organism. In some cases, surgical removal of the offending organism is required. This is the case when the organism creates a "shell" around the area of infection that effectively keeps the antibiotics from reaching the organism.

Tumors in the brain can cause chronic weakness if they occur in the area of the brain that is associated with the movement of muscles. Some tumors grow very slowly and can cause a gradual weakness that takes years to develop. These are usually benign tumors that don't spread to other parts of the body nor to other parts of the brain. They exert their influence on the movement associated wires of the brain by compressing and squashing them as the tumor grows, taking up more and more space within the non-expandable skull as it gets larger and larger. Malignant, faster growing tumors exert their influence on the normal brain in the same way, but they cause the weakness to appear and progress faster, over a period of weeks rather than years.

The treatment for tumors is surgical removal, in the case of the benign tumors, or radiation therapy, in the case of the faster growing, more invasive malignant tumors.

Radiation therapy involves the aiming of an X-ray beam at the area of the brain where the tumor is located. The X-ray beam disrupts the process of division of cells, and so any cell that happens to be dividing when the beam hits it dies. Tumors, especially the rapidly growing ones, contain almost all rapidly dividing cells, which is why they grow so fast. This rapid division makes them more susceptible to being killed by the X-ray beam. The wires that make up the brain are also cells, although very modified for carrying electric current, but they do not ever divide once they are formed. Because of this lack of division, they are thus protected from the harmful effects of the X-ray beam used for radiation therapy. The faster growing malignant tumors also have a tendency to send out little finger-like projections throughout the brain which makes them almost impossible to remove completely with surgery. The benign tumors are more rounded and easier to remove in total with surgery.

Multiple sclerosis is a disease that involves the insulation on the wires of the nerves within the brain. For unknown reasons, the white blood cells in a patient with multiple sclerosis begin attacking the insulation in small, isolated areas of the brain. It is as if the white blood cells think that the insulation on the wires in these areas is actually an invading group of germs that must be stopped. Any part of the brain is susceptible to these attacks and if the area involved happens to include the wires related to moving muscles, then the person with multiple sclerosis will become weak in the area of the body that corresponds to the area of the brain affected because this area of the brain can no longer send electric signals to the peripheral wires and then out to the muscles.

The treatment for the acute attacks of multiple sclerosis includes medications that slow down the production of white blood cells or inhibits their reactivity with the insulation on the wires in the brain. Medications that slow down the production of the white blood cells include the chemotherapy agents, azathioprine and cyclophosphamide. A medication that inhibits the reactivity of the white blood cells with the insulation on the wires of the brain is prednisone, which is usually given in very high doses each day for about one to two weeks.

Depression, as mentioned in the beginning of this chapter, is one of the most common causes of weakness. This can be for two different reasons. First, when someone is depressed for external reasons, such as the death of someone close to the person, the brain is occupied with electrical activity that centers around the emotional areas of the brain, stimulating memories associated with the person who has died. It is therefore more difficult to direct an electric current towards the areas of the brain associated with movement, which the person perceives as a weakness. This is not actually a malfunction of the wires associated with movement, but rather a "concentration" difficulty. (Remember from the chapters on memory and confusion that concentration is the directing of electric current towards an area of the brain that we wish to use at that particular time, whether for retrieving a memory, making a specific movement, such as fingering the keyboard of a guitar while playing a new tune that has not been committed to memory, or for determining the texture of an object that our fingers may be touching at that particular time.) In these cases, the "weakness" resolves when the depression is gone, or when the brain is able to direct electric current more easily to other areas of the brain besides the emotional areas.

The second way that depression can cause weakness is related to an intrinsic cause for the depression. That is, depression that is caused by a "chemical imbalance" within the brain, rather than from an external cause, such as mentioned above. The chemicals referred to in this case are the ones used to transfer the electric current from one wire within the brain to another wire within the brain. (Remember that the wires in the nervous system don't make direct contact with each other but have minute spaces between them. When an electric current gets to the end of a wire, it triggers these chemicals contained at the end of the wire to be released into the space between the wires. When the chemical diffuses across the space and touches the next wire, it starts the electric current flowing in that wire.) If the specific chemicals used to convey the electric current from one wire to the next are not at the proper concentrations, then the impulse doesn't get transmitted properly, if at all. If this occurs between two wires that are involved in the ultimate movement of muscles, then a feeling of weakness will result. In this case, the term

107

"depression" is probably not the best choice of words to explain the process, since although depression may occur with a chemical imbalance, it is not actually the "cause" of the weakness, only an associated symptom.

The treatment for both internal and external depression as a cause of generalized weakness is anti-depressants. There are many different ones on the market but all of them either replace one or both of two different chemicals that may be "out of balance". These are serotonin and norepinephrine.

Blood vessel malformations in the brain can also cause weakness if they are located in such an area that they either deprive the movement wires of blood and nutrients or compress the movement wires like a tumor. They consist of bunches of twisted, malformed blood vessels that shunt blood to other areas besides where the blood would normally go, thus depriving certain areas of an adequate blood supply. In some cases, they become so large that they can actually compress the brain that lies beneath or beside them. Their constant pulsations with every heartbeat also can do damage to the neighboring areas of the brain. Most of the damage they do to the brain is derived from their shunting of blood away from parts of the brain rather than from the compression of the brain by their occasionally large size. They occur as "birth defects" usually, but can also occur with trauma to the brain. When they shunt blood away from the wires involved with movement of muscles, weakness results. This is usually a localized, rather than generalized, weakness.

The treatment for blood vessel malformations depends on their location. If they are located on the surface of the brain, as they usually are, they can be removed with surgery. If they are located deeper in the substance of the brain, they are usually not operable and the person has to live with the symptoms. In some cases, a type of "glue" has been injected into the main blood vessel in the malformation in hopes of plugging it up and stopping the shunting of blood away. However, this procedure has produced some major problems when the glue travels downstream before it hardens, causing strokes.

Genetic defects in the brain can also cause weakness, usually of a generalized type, and usually occurring in children. Essentially all of these are of the "inborn errors of metabolism" type, or "storage" diseases. That is, the person lacks the ability to convert one substance to another in the long chain of reactions that take place within the brain cells to convert nutrients into energy and cell parts, and this leads to an accumulation of the substance that can't be converted within the brain cells. As the cell fills up with this substance and there is no more room left within the cell, that cell eventually dies. If the cell that dies happens to be one that is involved in muscle movement, then the person will begin showing signs of weakness. Although there are some of these genetic diseases that seem to affect only the wires of the brain associated with movement, the overwhelming majority affect many parts of the brain at the same time, causing other symptoms as well as weakness. These diseases caused by genetic defects are all rare and are not treatable, for the most part.

Most of the diseases mentioned above as chronic causes of weakness arising within the brain can also occur within the brainstem or the spinal cord.

PERIPHERAL NERVOUS SYSTEM

In the peripheral nervous system, there are also acute and chronic causes of weakness. All of these causes for weakness occur because of malfunctions in the peripheral wires between the spinal cord, where they begin, and the muscles, where they end. We will first discuss the acute causes of weakness, and then the chronic causes.

Chapter 7

ACUTE WEAKNESS OF PERIPHERAL
NERVOUS SYSTEM ORIGIN

Guillain-Barre disease usually occurs after a viral infection, following either a cold or flu. It is also sometimes called "ascending paralysis" because its symptoms, which consist of progressive weakness, usually start in both legs and then spread upward to the arms. The diaphragm, which is also a muscle, can be affected by this disease, and when it is, the person has to be placed on a ventilator as he or she is not able to breathe without assistance. The location of this disease is in the area of the peripheral wires just after they leave the spinal cord, and it usually only affects the wires that are used for moving muscles. The insulation on these wires gets attacked by the body's white blood cells, probably as a secondary effect of their action on the cold or flu virus. This is called an autoimmune disease because it is the result of our own immune system attacking a part of our bodies. Multiple sclerosis, mentioned above, is also an autoimmune disease.

There are a few theories on why our own immune system may attack our own bodies. The one that is most likely is that when a virus invades our body, the white blood cells recognize certain parts of the outside coat on the virus that the white blood cell can attach to in order to kill the virus. Sometimes, the outside coat on the virus is similar enough to the outside covering of various groups of our own cells such that the white blood cells cannot tell the difference between what is virus and what is "us". It ends up attacking everything that "looks" alike. (The reason the white blood cells don't attack our cells normally is because there are not enough of them to do any damage. But when a virus comes along, that stimulates the white blood cells to multiply to the point where there are huge numbers of them to fight off the viruses, and just because of the large numbers of them alone, some of them are likely to attach to and destroy cells whose coats look similar to the viruses, which they do.)

Guillain-Barre disease usually requires hospitalization because the weakness that results is usually severe. It can last for several months, but in most cases, it does get better.

Compression of various peripheral wires can also cause acute weakness. The most common areas where the wires can become compressed are the same areas as mentioned in the previous chapter on numbness and tingling. That is, in the arm, the wrist and the elbow are the most common areas where these "pressure palsies" occur. In the leg, the outside part of the knee is where they usually occur. Treatment for these causes of weakness is surgery. The surgeon usually will move the wire away from the bone that is causing the compression of that wire. The results of this surgical release are usually quite good.

Bell's palsy is an interesting phenomenon that occurs in the muscles of the face. It consists of paralysis of one half of the facial muscles such that the person who is afflicted with it is unable to close the eye on that side of the face, cannot move the affected side of the mouth, which droops down, and when he or she smiles, only the unaffected side of the mouth turns up. Since the person is unable to control the mouth movements on the affected side, when he or she attempts to eat, the food falls out of the mouth. Occasionally, a pain will be felt behind the ear on the affected side, and the person may not be able to taste food on the affected side. All of these symptoms are caused because the bundle of wires that goes to each half of the face, each of which includes wires that sense pain behind the ear and wires that go to the tongue for tasting, as well as the wires for moving the various muscles of that half of the face, has been compressed against the inner edge of the skull where it travels in a small groove, or tunnel, before it exits from the skull to go to the tongue, the muscles of the face, and to the area behind the ear. When this nerve swells up for one reason or another, usually as a side effect of a cold or flu-like illness, the nerve becomes compressed against the skull to the point where it can no longer function properly, resulting especially in the paralysis of one half of the face. The interesting part of this phenomenon is that although a Bell's palsy resembles a stroke with the classically droop-ing face, a stroke does not cause paralysis of the upper half of the face, and the person with a stroke is able to close the eye normally on the affected side. This makes it very easy to distinguish between the relatively benign Bell's palsy and the more serious stroke. The reason that a stroke does not cause paralysis of the upper half of the face is simply because in the brain, both upper halves of the face are rep-resented in both halves of the brain. Therefore, when a stroke occurs on one side of the brain in the area that affects the upper half of the face, the other uninvolved side of the brain can "take over" and move the muscles of the upper face normally. This double representation does not apply to the peripheral wires, however, which is why a Bell's palsy affects both the upper and lower half of the face. (It is not known why the upper half of the face is represented in both halves of the brain while the other parts of the face and the rest of the body are not.) The treatment for Bell's palsy is steroids over a short period of time and at high doses if the symptoms are present for less than a day or two. Once the bundle of wires has swelled up and paraly-sis is complete, even steroids won't help to restore the proper functioning of the wires. Fortunately, Bell's palsy usually cures itself over a period of about two months. Younger people do better with Bell's palsy than older peo-ple, who are more prone to have at least some residual weakness from the disease.

CHRONIC WEAKNESS OF PERIPHERAL NERVOUS SYSTEM ORIGIN

The most common cause of chronic weakness that is due to malfunction in the peripheral nervous system is medications. In fact, when I am asked to see patients who have a complaint of generalized weakness, the first thing I ask them is what medications they are taking. This often makes the diagnosis, especially with patients who are on several different medications that alone may not be offensive, but in combination with each other, can cause weakness. Medications work on the body in so many different ways that it would be difficult to determine how each actually causes weakness, and even more difficult to determine how the interactions of various medications can cause weakness.

The treatment for weakness caused by medications is to attempt to switch the patient to a similar, but less offensive, medication. Sometimes this is not possible. In these cases, it has to be determined whether the weakness or the need for the medication is more important to the patient, and then treat accordingly. Unfortunately, the choice that gives the most immediate results is frequently elected by the patient, which is not always the right choice. For instance, if someone is on blood pressure medication that is also making him or her weaker, the person may elect to stop the medication and will notice an improvement in strength. However, several weeks or months down the road, as the blood pressure begins to climb higher and higher without the patient's knowledge of this, he or she may ultimately suffer a stroke.

A kind of subset of medications as a cause for weakness is metabolic abnormalities. This refers to a lack, or excess, of certain elements in the person's body. The reference to this as a subset of medications as a cause of weakness is made because most of the metabolic abnormalities occur as a side effect of various medications. When a person's potassium level falls too low, or the calcium or magnesium levels rise too high, weakness can result. There are several medications that can deplete the body of potassium, the most common of which are the diuretics used for blood pressure control. Some antacids and laxatives contain magnesium and calcium, and chronic use of these can result in too much of these two elements in the body, which then results in weakness of a generalized nature.

Vitamins B12 and E can be used in the body to help convert various nutrients into energy. When these two vitamins are depleted from the body, a generalized weakness can result. Vitamin B12 is absorbed from a specific part of the intestines. Some people are unable to absorb this vitamin from the intestines and have a chronic shortage of it. This is especially true in people who have had surgery for removal of part of their intestines because of cancer or other problems. In these cases the vitamin B12 has to be given as an injection into the muscle in order to be absorbed.

Glucose is the main substance used by the body for energy. There are many systems in the body for converting various things that we eat into glucose for use as a direct energy source. When the glucose level falls in the blood, weakness, among other symptoms, always occurs. The weakness that results, as well as any weakness that is the result of various medications or metabolic problems, is of a generalized nature.

The next two causes of chronic weakness that results from peripheral nervous system origin are unique in that the first, amyotrophic lateral sclerosis (ALS), or Lou Gehrig's disease, affects the beginning, or origin of the peripheral wires where they connect to the spinal cord, and the second, myasthenia gravis, affects the very ends of the peripheral wires where they connect to the muscles.

ALS is a disease that results in the destruction of the

beginning parts of the peripheral wires that are used for moving muscles such that they are unable to receive electrical signals from the spinal cord. Although the cause for the destruction of the beginning portions of these wires is not known for sure, the most likely cause is a predetermined, abnormal program in the genetic code that causes this area of the peripheral wires for movement of muscles to shut down at some time in middle to late adulthood. There is no cure for this cause of chronic weakness, and there is no medication available to alleviate any of the symptoms.

Myasthenia gravis affects the other end of the peripheral wire where it attaches to the muscle. It causes the tip of the wire to become non-functional such that when an electric current travels down the wire, it stops when it reaches this point rather than being transmitted from the end of the wire to the surface of the muscle. This disease is caused by an autoimmune reaction as explained earlier. That is, a virus or other organism probably gets into the body, which causes the white blood cells to respond to it by increasing their numbers. If the invading organism happens to resemble the ends of the peripheral wires, which is assumed to occur in this case, the huge numbers of white blood cells may end up attacking the ends of the wires as well as attacking the invading organisms. This somehow becomes a self-perpetuating process which results in continued attacking of the peripheral wires by the white blood cells even after the offending organism is eliminated, resulting in the recurring weakness associated with this disease. It may also be the case that the problem is genetic in nature, as in ALS, and has nothing to do with invading organisms. At this point, no one knows for sure.

The treatment for myasthenia gravis includes various methods of decreasing the numbers of white blood cells. As with multiple sclerosis, steroids in high doses are used to decrease the reactivity of the white blood cells themselves, or the products they produce that interact in an adverse way with the wires. The chemotherapy agents azathioprine and cyclophosphamide are used to decrease the numbers of white blood cells by inhibiting their replication. There is another method of dealing with the chemicals produced by the white blood cells that also attack the ends of the wires, and that are continuously floating around in the blood after they are released from certain white blood cells. This method of ridding the body of these chemicals is called plasmapheresis. It consists of running the blood through a bath of agents that selectively removes these chemicals from the blood.

Another type of treatment for myasthenia gravis involves giving a medication that replaces the chemical that is released from the ends of the peripheral wires to stimulate the muscles to contract, as the disease causes this chemical to be in short supply. This medication is called pyridostigmine and it usually works quite well.

MUSCLE WEAKNESS

The final location for a source of weakness is in the muscles themselves. First we will discuss acute causes for muscle weakness, and then we will discuss the chronic causes.

Acute muscle weakness is usually due to either trauma, which is usually fairly obvious, or myositis, which is inflammation of the muscles themselves.

Myositis occurs for various reasons, including viral infections, side effects of various medications, and poor circulation to the muscles. The usual symptoms of myositis include a generalized weakness, which does not distinguish this disease from other causes of generalized weakness, and pain in the muscles, especially when they are squeezed, which does distinguish this cause for muscle weakness from the other forms of generalized weakness.

The treatment for myositis includes steroids, such as prednisone, or anti-inflammatory medications, such as ibuprofen and indomethicin.

Chronic muscle weakness is usually the result of genetic diseases and is usually seen early in life. There are several types of muscular dystrophy and all of them are hereditary. They may start in infancy with what is called "floppy baby syndrome" in which the infant has very poor muscle tone. Duchenne's muscular dystrophy is the most well known of these diseases as it is the type referred to in the various telethons that are presented on television. It is first noted in early childhood and usually results in death because of inability to contract the diaphragm for breathing by the early 20's. There is no treatment for any of these causes for chronic muscle weakness.

Another more common cause of chronic muscle weakness is disuse atrophy. This occurs in people who are bedridden because of other medical problems, usually. When a muscle is not used for even a short period of time, such as a week or two, there will be a noticeable decrease in the size of the muscle because of atrophy. This is seen frequently in the hospital in patients who have been hospitalized for a few weeks. When they are medically able to be discharged from the hospital, they find that they are no longer able to walk because of disuse atrophy of the leg muscles. Now, most patients who are in the hospital for longer than a few days are automatically treated by the physical therapy departments to prevent this problem from occurring.

GUARDING

There is one last category of weakness that is not really a weakness at all, but is perceived as a weakness. This is weakness that is the result of pain that occurs when moving a specific body part. This is also called "guarding" and consists of protecting the body part from moving to avoid the pain that is associated with its movement. There is nothing actually malfunctioning in the central or peripheral nervous system that deals with movement of muscles, and there is nothing wrong with the muscles themselves, but the person who has pain with movement will usually say that he or she is "weak". The most common cause of guarding is arthritis. Treatment for this cause of "weakness" includes anti-inflammatory medications.

In summation, there are many causes for weakness, some of which are fairly benign and some of which are fairly serious. If one remembers, however, that 95% of all weakness is related either to medications or depression, if generalized in nature, and stroke, if localized to one side of the body and not associated with pain, it becomes much easier to determine the cause of the weakness and at least alleviate some of the anxiety about it.

Chapter 8
TREMORS AND OTHER ABNORMAL MOVEMENTS

In the previous chapter on weakness, the main wires that run directly from the cortex of the brain down through the brainstem, the spinal cord, the peripheral wires, and then finally to the muscles, were discussed. As the current flows through all of these different areas, it can be modified by the influence of current in other wires along the way, which was not previously mentioned since it does not directly pertain to "weakness". In this chapter, we will discuss what happens when these modifiers of the current that moves muscles malfunction. In some cases, when these modifiers malfunction, the result is a tremor of the body part that is involved. In other cases, wild, flinging movements or slow, writhing movements might result. The most common symptom that results, however, is a tremor, usually of the hands or arms.

We will also discuss causes of tremors that don't originate in the modifiers of the current that is used to move muscles. However, these causes of tremors are very rare in comparison to malfunctions that occur in the modifiers of electric current used for moving muscles.

Most tremors originate from malfunctions in the sub-cortical areas, including the brainstem and the cerebellum. The brainstem contains several areas that exert influence upon wires that carry information from the cortex of the brain to the muscles for movement. The cerebellum, which is a small pocket of brain tissue that sits below the cortex and behind the brainstem, has always been thought of as the main modulator of movement so that all our movements are very smooth in nature rather than jerking.

As the current to move a muscle originates in the cortex of the brain, then begins its course through the brainstem, some of the current "forks" off onto wires from the brainstem and cerebellum that are attached to the main movement wire. This electrical current that forks off can become amplified or reduced in the brainstem or cerebellum, then returns to the main movement wire a very short time later. As this process of amplifying and reducing the current occurs in several thousand different areas along the course of the movement wire, the original crude impulse generated by the cortex of the brain becomes very sophisticated to the point where extremely delicate movements, such as threading a needle, can be performed. Without this modification of the original impulse generated in the movement area of the cortex of the brain, we would be unable to perform a task as simple as picking up a glass of water without spilling it all over. We would also be unable to judge how tightly to grip a paper cup such that we would probably end up crushing it and spilling whatever was inside.

As alluded to in the crushing of a paper cup without the influence of the modifiers as mentioned above, the sensory system is also involved when performing a task with the muscles. Information has to be constantly sent back to the brainstem modifiers in the way of electrical current on sensory wires to help the brainstem (and cerebellum) modify the movement current in the proper way such that a paper cup, for example, is not gripped too tightly. What happens because of all this interaction of sensory input and modifier action in the brainstem is that a single, short, crude, impulse triggered in the cortex of the brain to pick up a cup, for example, becomes a long, continuous series of electrically modified impulses running together and in a sequence that results in a smooth continuous action by the muscles involved to pick up the cup in a very smooth fashion. This system normally works very well and doesn't require any voluntary effort on our part to keep it functioning. The only voluntary part of the whole system is the initial signal that is generated in the cortex of the brain to start the whole process of the ultimate movement of a muscle or group of muscles.

All of the various areas in the brainstem and the cerebellum that are used for modulating movements are normally only active when there is a movement signal generated by the cortex of the brain to act upon. One would expect, then, that malfunctions of these areas of the brainstem and cerebellum would only be noticed when movements are attempted. In general, this is the case. However, there are instances where malfunctions can cause these areas to generate their own movement type electric currents, resulting in what are called "resting" tremors. These are tremors that occur even when a person is not trying to move any specific muscles. That is, there is no voluntary electric signal being generated in the movement area of the cortex of the brain for the brainstem and cerebellum to act upon, but these two areas generate their own abnormal electric signals, which continue in an abnormal continuous circuit, over and over, creating the rhythmic movement of the body part involved.

Tremors can occur gradually over a long period of time or can be fairly abrupt, or acute, in onset. We will first discuss the acute causes for tremor and will then discuss the chronic causes.

ACUTE TREMOR

The most common cause for acute onset of tremor is a stroke in the brainstem or cerebellum. The blood supply to the brainstem and cerebellum is not as good as it is in many other parts of the brain and, consequently, these areas are more prone to strokes. If a stroke occurs in one area of the brainstem, the patient may exhibit a resting tremor, while, if the stroke occurs in a different area of the brainstem, he or she may exhibit flinging type movements of the arms, or writhing, slow, wormlike movements. The type movements or tremors that are seen can help localize where the actual stroke has occurred, even without the aid of a CAT scan or MRI scan of the brain, in many cases.

Epilepsia partialis continua is a type of seizure in which a constant tremor of one arm persists. The patient is awake throughout the entire seizure but cannot stop his or her arm or hand from shaking. This tremor can go on for days at a time if it is not treated. It is seen in diabetics and is caused by a blood glucose level greater than 300, usually. Not every diabetic who has a glucose greater than 300 will develop this seizure type, but those who are prone to it will invariably get it when their glucose reaches this level. It usually doesn't spread to involve any other extremities, even when it persists for several hours or days. If an electroencephalogram (EEG) is performed, the seizure activity will be seen originating in the part of the cortex of the brain that controls movement in the tremulous arm. It appears very much like a "standard" tremor, but starts fairly abruptly and is confined to one arm and hand only. The treatment for this is to lower the glucose level by administering insulin. This usually will abolish the seizure activity in the brain, as well as the associated visible tremor, fairly quickly. There is no need to give the patient any seizure medications, and they usually don't work for this type of tremor anyway. This phenomenon is relatively rare in diabetics and is often missed when trying to determine the cause for an acute tremor that occurs in one arm.

Psychogenic tremor is a voluntary tremor which is usually not too difficult to diagnose because of the rate and amplitude of the tremor. That is, the oscillations of the rhythmic movements of the tremor are not constant. Sometimes the tremor will be fast in frequency, and at other times it will be slow. The amplitude of the tremor will vary as well. Sometimes the tremor will be exaggerated and at other times it may be less obvious. The tremor will disappear when asking the person to concentrate on one task while doing something else with the tremulous body part. The tremor also disappears when no one else is around.

The most common cause for a psychogenic tremor is impending litigation. People who have been involved in auto accidents and work related injuries are more likely to develop psychogenic tremor than anyone else, and their tremors seem to disappear once their cases are settled.

Medications can also cause a relatively acute tremor. This type tremor is usually a fine rather than exaggerated, or course tremor, and involves the arms and hands moreso than the legs and feet. The head is often involved as well. Many of the anti-depressants and seizure medications can be associated with a tremor such as this. Some of the medications used for the symptoms associated with colds and flu can also cause a tremor.

Medication withdrawal is an important cause for tremor. All of the addictive, or habit forming, medications can cause tremor if they are suddenly discontinued. This is because of the way in which they act upon the brain. That is, when they enter the blood stream and are carried to the brain where they can interact with the brain tissue, they cause a decrease in the activity of the wires of the brain.

Since the brain is designed to always have a certain level of activity in the various wires, it compensates for this decrease in activity by producing more of the chemicals that stimulate the various wires in the brain. It also grows more branches on the ends of the wires to connect with other wires in the area so that, instead of one ending of a wire connecting with the beginning of the next wire, there might be 5 or 6 ends on the one wire to connect with the beginning of the next wire to make up for the decrease of electrical activity that results from using the medication. Then, when the medication is suddenly discontinued and there is no longer anything hindering the electric current in the wires of the brain, the excess chemicals that were produced in response to the medication, as well as the excess growth of ends on the wires, cause the wires in the brain to become overactive. This, then, produces too much current in the wires of the brain, and is manifested as the withdrawal tremor.

Although most of the addictive pain medications cause this phenomenon, as do the benzodiazepines, which include all of the members of the valium family, such as many of the anti-anxiety agents and sleeping aids (librium, xanax, klonopin, restoril, dalmane, halcion, ativan, and others), the most well known offender is alcohol. This is why chronic alcoholics are "nervous", or tremulous, until they can get a drink, when they have gone for an extended period of time without alcohol.

Sydenham's chorea is an abnormal movement disorder that is seen in some children who have contracted a strep infection prior to the development of the abnormal movements. These consist of contortions of the face and hands in slow, writhing type movements which are usually quite upsetting to the parents. The movements of the face appear to be almost voluntary in nature and, in fact, many children are reprimanded for "making faces" before they are finally diagnosed with this syndrome. A blood test is performed to check for ASO titers, which measures the body's immune response to a strep infection, and if this titer is high, then there is no doubt that the child has Sydenham's chorea. The treatment consists of antibiotics for the strep infection, usually for several years to prevent the heart problems that can be associated with this type infection, and haloperidol is used to control the abnormal movements when they are severe. Haloperidol decreases some of the electric current in the wires of the brain, thus decreasing the abnormal movements.

CHRONIC TREMOR

The most common cause of gradually increasing tremors is hardening of the arteries of the brainstem and cerebellum with passing time. As the arteries fill up with calcium deposits and other "junk", they become less able to carry an appropriate amount of nutrients to the various parts of the brainstem and cerebellum, which causes a gradual decrease in their ability to function properly. In a way, this can be thought of as a form of tiny strokes that accumulate over the years, since a stroke results from lack of blood supply to a part of the brain. Because of the nature of this type cause for tremors, other parts of the brain are affected as well, and one usually sees many other symptoms besides tremor in these cases, including difficulty with balance, lightheadedness when first getting up from a sitting to a standing position, dementia, and stiffness in the muscles.

Parkinson's disease is fairly well known, and although it consists of many symptoms, the one most often thought of as the hallmark of Parkinson's disease is the "resting tremor" that is observed. This is a deliberate, slow movement of an arm or hand that is often referred to as a "pill rolling tremor" which is present even when the person with Parkinson's disease is not trying to perform some task with that particular arm or hand. There has been much research done on this disease. It has been known for a long time which part of the brainstem malfunctions to cause the symptoms of Parkinson's disease. It is one of the causes of tremor mentioned near the beginning of this chapter that results not from abnormal modification of a signal that originates from one of the movement wires of the cortex of the brain, but rather, from an abnormal production of current on its own that travels to the arm or hand, for example, from a continuously repeating circuit in the brainstem, over and over, which produces the continuous, repetitive movements of the hand or arm.

The cause for Parkinson's disease is a lack of a specific chemical in a specific area of the brainstem that helps with controlling smooth movements of various muscle groups. The treatment for Parkinson's disease usually consists of a medication to replace the one that is in short supply as a result of the disease. This chemical is called "dopamine" and is able to be reproduced and given as a pill. There are other pills that, rather than acting as a replacement for the decreased levels of dopamine, work by causing more dopamine to be made available for use by the wires. There have been experiments performed where tissue is implanted into the brain that is purported to continuously replace the dopamine that is lacking in Parkinson's disease, but there have been some ethical questions raised about using this tissue as it is derived from fetuses.

An action tremor is one that occurs only when attempting to voluntarily move a specific body part. It is the result of the modifiers of a movement signal that originates in the cortex of the brain exerting an abnormal influence on that signal such that a smooth movement of the muscle group involved does not occur. When the arm or leg, for example, is in the resting position, there is no tremor because there are no signals being generated by the cortex of the brain to be acted upon by the abnormal signal modifiers in the brainstem. This type of tremor usually gets worse with advancing age. This would suggest a cause associated with the aging process, such as hardening and subsequent occlusion of the arteries which results in decreased or absent blood flow to these parts of the brain-stem. This is known to actually be the case in many of these types of tremors.

An action tremor becomes more pronounced when the person with this problem is anxious, under stress, or emotionally taxed while trying to perform some move-ment. This is because with anxiety, stress, or emotion, there is more electrical current being generated in the brain by the areas responsible for these three states. This extra cur-rent can also modify the primary movement signals that are generated in the cortex of the brain, and is generated by an increase in one of the chemicals released at the ends of one wire that then causes the current to spread to the beginning point of the next wire so that it can continue to flow. When there is too much of this chemical in the spaces between the wires, then there are too many wires stimulat-ed to carry current, and the tremor becomes much more pronounced. The chemical in this case is a form of adrena-lin.

Familial tremor is a type of action tremor that is inherited. It can start as early as the teenage years and is progressive with time. What usually causes a person to seek out the help of a neurologist when afflicted with a familial tremor is a difficulty with writing. The patients' penmanship can become so poor that banks won't recog-nize the signature and refuse to honor checks written on their accounts.

The treatment for the various tremors caused by mal-functions in the brainstem includes medications that block the release of the chemicals from the ends of the wires that allow the current to spread to the next wire in the sequence, thus decreasing the overall amount of current in the system, and theoretically, the amount of tremor. Some blood pressure medications, such as propranolol, work well in this regard. (These medications control blood pressure by the same mechanism.)

Clonazepam, which is a member in the valium family of medications, also works to control tremor to some degree. It works by stimulating wires that are used by the nervous system for actually decreasing electric current. (Until now, there has been no mention of any wires that decrease electrical activity in the nervous system when they are activated, but they exist, nevertheless. They are used, along with the other types of wires already mentioned, to help "mold" a crude signal generated somewhere in the brain into a "smoother" signal. There are probably as many of these "inhibitory" wires as there are "excitatory" wires in the nervous system.) It may seem odd that a wire that carries an electric current can actually decrease an electric current, but in this case, the way that inhibitory wires decrease the current traveling down another wire is by attaching to that wire somewhere other than at the very end, such that it can send current up the wire it attaches to. When the current traveling up the wire meets the current traveling down the wire, they cancel each other out, and the current stops flowing for the most part. Clonazepam is one of the medications that increases the activity in these inhibitory wires, effectively decreasing the abnormal activity being generated, in the brainstem in this case, that may be causing a tremor.

Cerebellar tremor originates in the area of the brain that is below the cortex and behind the brainstem. The most usual cause of a cerebellar tremor is a stroke in this area of the brain. Cerebellar tremors are always action type tremors. That is, they don't occur unless a person is trying to move a part of the body. They don't occur while a person is sleeping or at rest. There is also no treatment for a cerebellar tremor as it does not respond to any of the medications mentioned above.

Asterixis is a very crude type tremor that occurs when someone has a profound liver disease. What occurs with this type of abnormal movement is a complete loss of muscle tone in a muscle group, such as in an arm or a leg, for less than a second. If, for instance, a person is holding his arm out, it will suddenly begin dropping, then correct itself once the loss of tone is passed. As this occurs over and over, it resembles a crude tremor. The treatment for this is correction of the liver problem, if this is able to be done. Usually, however, by the time a person develops asterixis, the liver is too diseased to recover.

Clonus can be thought of as a type of tremor that occurs when there is a loss of inhibitory input from the brain upon the reflexes, usually in the ankle. When a normal reflex occurs, such as when tapping on a person's knee with a reflex hammer, an electric impulse is generated by the stretching of the mechanoreceptors in the knee. This electric sensory impulse then travels to the spinal cord and then to both the brain and directly to a movement wire located in the spinal cord which causes the leg to "jump" almost immediately. This "jumping" of the leg then stretches the mechanoreceptor in the knee again and the cycle would be repeated over and over if it weren't for the influence of the brain, which sends an electric signal down the spinal cord that interrupts the circuit mentioned above by sending current in the opposite direction to cancel the incoming impulse from the mechanoreceptor in the knee and stops the jerking of the leg. When a patient has a malfunction of the system such that the impulse does not get sent to the brain, but only back to the spinal cord, such as occurs when someone is paralyzed from a broken neck, for example, clonus occurs and the ankle or knee continues to oscillate until it is extended, which will stop this action, usually.

To summarize, most tremors originate because of

malfunctions in the modifiers of movement signals that originate in the cortex of the brain. These modifiers of the movement signals are located in the brainstem and in the cerebellum. The most common cause of tremors is decreased blood flow to these areas of the brain from natural aging processes as well as the effects of chronic high blood pressure and other diseases that affect the circulation system. Other causes of tremors were discussed, but these are much less common.

Chapter 9
NECK AND BACK PAIN

The most common cause of missed days from work is neck pain and back pain. I would estimate that 35 to 40% of the patients that I see in my office give neck or back pain as the reason for their visits. There are so many different ways that a person can injure his or her neck or back that it is often difficult to establish an exact cause for a specific neck or back pain. As with many of the neurologic diseases mentioned so far, there are both acute and chronic forms of neck and back pain. The origins for the acute forms are usually easier to determine because of a cause and effect situation, such as low back pain that occurs when a person wakes up after he or she had been moving furniture the previous day. It is more difficult to determine the origin of the chronic forms since there may or may not be an acute cause for a neck or back pain that seems to recur over and over on days that seem to be particularly worse than others.

Over 95% of neck and back pain, in my experience, is caused by one or more of three distinct malfunctions in the tissues of the neck or back. These include muscle spasms of the neck or back, bone spurs, either in or on the spine, and disk malfunctions. Statistically, about 80% of the time, the cause is muscle spasms. The rest of the 20% is about evenly divided among bone spurs in the spine, degeneration of the disks between the bones of the spine, and bulging or herniated disks. We will discuss each of these causes for neck and back pain, and then we will discuss the less common causes for the remaining few per cent after that.

MUSCLE SPASMS

In order to understand why muscle spasms can be so prevalent as a cause for neck or back pain, it is important to understand how the muscles of the neck and back work to convert nutrients into energy in order to function normally to support our bodies while in an upright position, such as while standing or sitting, as well as to balance our bodies when we lift or carry something.

There are three types of muscle tissue in our bodies. The first type is cardiac muscle, which is a special type of muscle only found in the heart. The second type is smooth muscle, which is the type found inside the intestines for moving food along by rhythmically contracting. It is also found inside of blood vessels that carry blood from the heart to the various tissues of the body, and is responsible for increasing or decreasing the diameter of the blood vessels to deliver more or less blood to various areas of the body. The third type, which is the only type that we are concerned with for purposes of this discussion, is skeletal muscle.

There are two types of skeletal muscle in our bodies. One type is used for quick movements of various muscle groups and is very inefficient in the way that it uses energy stores for the purpose of movement. The second type is used for slower, more sustained movements. This type of muscle tissue is much more efficient in its use of the energy stores available, and it is this efficiency of energy usage that creates the problems associated with neck or back spasms.

The muscles in our arms and legs are of the type that perform quicker movements and are less efficient. Instead of converting the nutrients that they use for energy all the way down to carbon dioxide and water by a long series of reactions that are relatively slow, they convert nutrients into intermediate by-products and a lesser amount of energy, but at a faster rate. These intermediate by-products then can accumulate in the muscle tissue if nutrients are burned up at a relatively fast rate, such as would occur in the legs when a person is running at a high rate of speed. As these intermediate by-products accumulate, they eventually "poison" the muscle tissue temporarily, until they can eventually be removed by the blood. In other words, these toxic by-products can be produced by the muscle faster than they can be removed from the muscle tissue by the blood. When this phenomenon occurs, the muscle becomes very painful until the toxic products are completely removed. More importantly, the relatively inefficient utilization of the energy stores in this way uses them up very fast, causing the muscle to be unable to continue contracting. The result is that the muscle relaxes. Later, after the energy stores have a chance to build back up again, and the toxic by-products, which consist mainly of lactic acid, are removed, the muscle is able to contract again.

The muscles of the neck and back are slow muscles. They don't convert nutrients to the by-products, such as lactic acid, mentioned above. Because they work at a relatively slow pace, the muscles of the neck and back are able to convert the nutrients used for contracting all the way down to carbon dioxide and water with no accumulation of other toxic by-products to temporarily poison the muscle. And because they are so efficient in their utilization of the nutrients, they don't burn them up as quickly as if they were converting them to intermediate by-products. This allows the blood to carry away the carbon dioxide before it is allowed to "poison" the muscles. The result of all this is that these slow muscles are able to maintain a sustained contraction almost indefinitely. When one thinks about it, this is important for the functioning of the neck and back muscles because at all times when we are in the sitting or standing position, these muscles must be in the contracted state continuously to keep us from falling over. It is ultimately this efficiency of the muscles that causes the problem with neck and back pain that occurs because of muscle spasms.

As mentioned earlier, muscle spasms of the neck or back can occur for a variety of reasons. Among these, trauma and stress are by far the most common causes. Other causes, such as the "crick" that develops in a person's neck or back from sleeping in an awkward position, muscle spasms that result from malformed backbones (scoliosis), or muscle spasms that result from walking with a limp due to a problem with a foot or leg which causes uneven pressure on the two sides of the back are less commonly seen.

Trauma does not usually "damage" a muscle. What usually occurs with trauma is that the muscle is stretched faster than it is designed to be stretched, and when this occurs, the muscle responds with an exaggerated contraction, or shortening, of the entire muscle for a period of time. If the muscle is stretched too fast or too far, it can actually tear. This almost never happens, however. Once the muscle contracts, or shortens, in response to being stretched too fast, it pinches the peripheral wires that have just exited from the spinal cord in these areas. (The peripheral wires pass through the long muscles located from the base of the skull all the way down to the lowest part of the back in order to get to where the wires are eventually going, in the arms and legs, for example, and when these muscles that the wires pass through contract, or shorten, they compress the wires.) When the peripheral wire becomes compressed by the abnormally contracting muscle, it sends a sensory impulse to the brain, making the brain aware of the abnormal compression of the wire. The brain interprets this compression of the peripheral wire as damage in that area of the spine and immediately sends a signal down a movement wire which contracts the muscles in that area for the purpose of immobilizing the spinal joints in that area so that further damage is not done. You see, the brain does not know whether the abnormal compression of the peripheral wire is due to a fracture of the spine or the simple muscle spasms, but the brain is "programmed" to treat all abnormal compressions of the peripheral nerves near the spine as potentially serious injuries, and therefore, tries to protect the area from being damaged further as would occur if an unstable fracture of the neck, for example, was allowed to move, such that the spinal cord could become severed. When the brain immobilizes the area by contracting all the muscles in that area so that the neck or back cannot be easily moved, it effectively puts that area in a muscle "splint" which, if a person actually had a fractured neck, may be the thing that protects them from ultimately severing the spinal cord and becoming paralyzed. Unfortunately, in the case of muscle spasms as a source of compression of the peripheral wires in the area in question, the brain's protective mechanism of contracting all the muscles in that area turns out to be a good system gone awry. That is, the brain effectively ends up causing the already excessively contracted back or neck muscles to contract even more. A vicious cycle results. The more the muscles contract, the more they compress the peripheral wires in that area, and the more they compress the peripheral wires in that area, the more the wires send sensory impulses to the brain, and the more the wires send sensory impulses to the brain, the more the brain sends movement signals back down the wires to contract the muscles even more, and the cycle continues over and over.

The result of all this is that the back or neck spasms become the source of a chronic pain in that area because they cannot resolve as long as the cycle mentioned above continues. This whole process can occur over a few days to a few weeks, depending on how severe the original trauma was.

One of the most difficult things about treating muscle spasms as a cause for neck or back pain is convincing a patient that this is indeed what the problem is. Most people wonder how they can be in so much pain if it's "only muscle spasms" in their necks or backs. In actuality, muscle spasms can cause much more severe pain than a ruptured disc or arthritic bone spurs. This is because muscle spasms are dynamic rather than static in nature. That is, muscle spasms don't simply contract to a certain point and then stay like that. They continually squeeze tighter and tighter, then relax a little, then squeeze down again. This constantly changing pressure on the peripheral wires is what causes such intense pain. It is because of the basic way that the brain handles incoming sensory information. If a wire keeps sending the same sensory signal over and over to the brain, the brain will stop responding to it after awhile. This is so that the brain doesn't get bogged down with extensive sensory information tying up all of the circuits in the brain. For example, when we first sit down on a chair, we are aware of the chair pressing against our bodies. As we sit there longer, eventually we don't feel the chair pressing against us. If we shift in our seat, however, then different mechanoreceptors begin sending information up the sensory wires to the brain and the brain begins paying attention to the incoming sensory information again for a short period of time. Pain signals work similar to this. That is, if the muscle spasms in the neck or back were to stay at the same level of tension, eventually the pain would diminish in severity because of the brain's tendency to disregard identical repeated incoming sensory signals after awhile. But when the muscle spasms keep changing in the amount of tension they are creating, the brain receives new information continuously from the pain wires that are being compressed by the muscle spasms, and the continued processing of this changing pain information is perceived by the brain as more intense pain than if the muscle tension remained the same. This is what usually makes neck or back spasms so much more painful than ruptured disks and bone spurs in the spine. When someone comes into my office with a complaint of neck or back pain, and is unable to sit still because of the pain, I am usually fairly confident that the pain is being produced by muscle spasms.

Usually, the diagnosis of muscle spasms can be made by examining a patient with symptoms of neck or back pain. Since almost all of neck and back pain is caused by either muscle spasms, bulging or ruptured disks, and bone spurs, then if there were a way to distinguish between these three causes of the pain, it would make the treatment much easier to plan. Normally, if a person has neck or back spasms, these can be felt by pressing in on the area of the neck or back that is causing the pain. Patients will often say that they have "knots" or "swollen areas" in their necks and backs. They may also have symptoms of "popping" of the neck or back when they turn their heads or bodies from one position to another. This "popping" is caused from the muscle spasms pulling the bones of the spine closer together such that they don't glide smoothly over one another as the person moves from one position to another, but instead, they have a tendency to grind together from the increased pressure.

The most commonly used treatment for muscle spasms is muscle relaxers, of which there are several. Most of these work by breaking up the vicious cycle of pain that results from the muscle spasms causing compression of the sensory wires, which then cause the brain to send impulses down the movement wires to compress the muscles even more. I have had the most success with baclofen, carisoprodol, and methocarbamol. None of these are considered to be habit-forming and have only limited side effects. In addition, methocarbamol can be given intravenously for faster relief from the muscle spasms. Heating pads, ultrasound treatments, and massage therapy sometimes help also. Pain killers do not have much use for giving resolution of neck and back spasms. They can mask the pain for a few hours, but do nothing to help abolish the cause of the pain and, since most of the prescription pain relievers have some type of addictive component to them, their continued use creates a second problem, this being addiction.

Muscle relaxers usually have to be taken for several weeks on a daily basis in order to abolish the muscle spasms permanently. It can sometimes be very difficult to convince patients of this. Also, muscle relaxers should be taken for several days after the pain has completely resolved or the muscle spasms have a tendency to return quickly. It seems that once a person has had muscle spasms of the neck or back, he or she is much more likely to have the spasms return with overexertion than someone who has never had back or neck spasms before. It is as if the pathway for the cycle of muscle spasms, sensory wires, and movement wires is always present once it has been established, and is just waiting for an opportunity to reestablish itself.

Besides the examination of the person with neck or back pain, there are a few tests that can be performed to determine whether a patient has muscle spasms or some other cause for the symptoms. These tests usually include an electromyogram, which consists of sending electric impulses up the various wires in the arms or legs until they reach the spinal cord. If the wires are being compressed by bone or cartilage, this test will show some abnormalities, whereas, if the wires are being compressed by muscle spasms, there will be no abnormalities seen. An MRI can also be done to give an actual picture of the bones and disks of the neck or back to determine whether an abnormality exists in either of these two tissues as a cause for the neck or back pain. If the MRI is normal, then by a process of elimination, the person's neck or back pain is most likely caused from muscle spasms. Myelograms were used frequently in the past to diagnose neck or back pain, but this test has been all but eliminated with the advent of the MRI, which is much more tolerable by patients. There are some cases, however, where the myelogram is used in order to better show the individual areas where the wires first exit from the spinal cord in order to see if the wire is being pinched between two bones. The myelogram is done by injecting a dye into the spinal canal. The dye outlines everything in the spinal canal, including disks, bone spurs, and the roots of the wires as they come off the spinal cord.

Most of the time, listening to how the patient developed neck or back pain, along with the examination of the patient, will usually allow making the correct diagnosis. If muscle spasms are strongly suspected as the cause of a patient's neck or back pain, based on the patient's history and examination, there is no need to perform any of the above mentioned tests which, by the way, are all relatively expensive. In these cases, one simply needs to take a muscle relaxer for a few weeks. It is also important to remember that, without any further information except that a person has neck pain or back pain, there is a 75 to 80% chance that the cause is muscle spasms.

An interesting phenomenon about muscle spasms of the neck or back is that if they start in the low back and nothing is done about them for awhile, they will usually spread to involve the neck as well. The reverse is also true when the spasms start in the neck. Also, if a person has chronic neck problems, he or she will almost certainly begin having associated headaches that start in the neck and radiate up over the top of the head and occasionally settle behind the eyes where they may cause the eyes to feel like there is a pressure behind them. All of this spreading of symptoms from one place to another is because of the fact that all the muscles of the neck and back are connected together and as one muscle contracts to the point where it develops into a spasm, it tends to "pull" the rest of the connected muscles into the spasm along with it over time. In the case of the headaches that result from muscle spasms, the muscles of the neck are attached to the scalp and as these muscles contract when they spasm, they pull on the scalp to cause the headache that radiates up over the top of the head.

BONE AND CARTILAGE

Since bone and cartilage cause neck and back pain in similar ways, they will be discussed together.

The most common cause of neck and back pain, second to muscle spasms of the neck and back, is degenerative disk disease.

The disks are soft cartilage "pillows" that lie in between each of the bones that make up the spine. They act as shock absorbers for the spine to prevent fractures of the bones of the spine when we run, jump, and especially when we fall. Over the years, with all the stress that can occur from lifting, twisting, walking, riding in cars, and supporting the weight of our bodies, the disks have a tendency to shrink in thickness. As this occurs, the bones that they separate are allowed to come closer together. Unfortunately, the wires that exit from the center of the spinal column pass through holes created between two successive bones of the spinal column, and when the disks become thinner with age, and the two bones that a particular disk separates become closer together because of this, the wires get pinched in between the two bones. This can result in chronic neck or back pain from these pinched peripheral wires. This whole process can produce a lot of swelling in the neck or back because of the chronic irritation of the tissues surrounding the bones and disks. This swelling adds to the problem by compressing, or pinching, the wires even more. Anti-inflammatory medications, such as ibuprofen and naproxen, as well as 30 or 40 others, can sometimes alleviate the symptoms, especially if the symptoms are mainly due to the swelling of the surrounding tissues rather than due to the actual compression of the wires by the bones themselves. If anti-inflammatory medications don't relieve the pain, then a bone surgeon or neurosurgeon may remove the part of the bone that is compressing the wires, thus making the hole that the wires pass through bigger. This is called a laminectomy.

Occasionally, bone spurs from arthritis can form in the area where the peripheral wires exit from the spine. If these bone spurs irritate the wires by pinching them, a pain in the neck or back will result. These are also treated in the same way as degenerative disk disease. That is, a conservative approach with anti-inflammatory medications is tried first in the hopes that most of the pain is due to the swelling of the tissues surrounding the bone spur. But if this doesn't work, then the bone spurs may need to be removed surgically.

A ruptured, or herniated, disk can occur spontaneously, especially in someone who is extremely obese, but this is relatively rare. Most ruptured disks are the result of trauma that is severe, such as would result from a fall of several feet onto the neck or back. (A ruptured disk is a condition where the disk material has actually been forced out of the sack-like container that keeps it in place in the spine.) It cannot be "pulled" back into place with traction, as can occasionally be done with a mildly bulging disk. The part of the disk that has ruptured usually has to be surgically removed, especially if it is compressing the peripheral wires in that area. In some cases, when there is not much of the disk left after removal of the ruptured part, and the two bones that were previously kept separated by that disk are then able to collapse together, the surgeon must put a brace in between the bones after he or she removes the disk in order to keep the peripheral wire from being permanently crushed between the bones.

Tests that are performed to diagnose a problem with a disk or the bones of the spine are the same as for diagnosing muscle spasms. These include the electromyogram, which is done by a neurologist in his or her office, and the MRI of the neck or back. Occasionally, a myelogram is performed, but, as stated earlier, these have been all but eliminated by the advent of the MRI, which is not as traumatic to the patient. These tests are fairly specific for diagnosing neck and back problems and make it relatively easy to find the cause of a person's source of pain.

We have now covered over 95% of the causes of neck and back pain. The remaining causes are subsequently more rare.

OTHER CAUSES

Occasionally, a person will develop a mass type lesion in the neck or back that will cause pain in that area because of the pressure it exerts, either on the back, the neck, or the peripheral wires. These mass type lesions can be in the form of tumors, cysts, blood vessel malformations, or infections. Although all of them are rare, the least rare of these is tumors that have spread from another place, such as from the prostate, the colon, or the lungs. Tumors that have spread to the neck or back from other places are usually quite ominous and signify a very poor chance of recovery.

Compression fractures can be seen, usually in the lower back area, almost exclusively in "little old ladies".

The cause of this problem is a lack of estrogen as women get older. Estrogen is a requirement for maintaining bone integrity and a lack of it causes the bones to become weak to the point where they will spontaneously "crack" under the weight of the person's body. The treatment for this is usually replacement estrogen and calcium but, unfortunately, this usually needs to be started long before the symptoms are actually present to be effective.

To summarize, about 75 to 80% of all neck and back pain is caused from muscle spasms of the neck or back. About 15 to 20% of neck and back pain is caused from bone and disk diseases. Diagnosing the cause of neck and back pain is fairly easy and involves getting a history of how the pain originated, examining the person, and in some cases, performing an electromyogram (EMG) or MRI of the neck or back. Essentially all neck and back pain can be accurately diagnosed in this way. Treatment consists of muscle relaxers most of the time, anti-inflammatory medications some of the time, and rarely, surgery.

Chapter 9

Chapter 10
SLEEP PROBLEMS

We spend about a third of our lives sleeping. We are not productive while we are sleeping, and if we don't get enough sleep on a particular night, we are usually not very productive the following day.

Sleep problems fall into two categories. People either complain when they are getting too much sleep or they complain when they are not getting enough sleep. The much more common complaint by far is of not getting enough sleep.

In this chapter, we will discuss insomnia, or a lack of sleep, and then we will discuss hypersomnia, or too much sleep. First, however, it is necessary to discuss what the sleep process is all about. That is, in order to understand what can go wrong with the sleep mechanism, it is important to know why we sleep at all, what takes place within the brain when we are asleep that cannot take place while we are awake, and the various stages of sleep that normally occur in a typical night's sleep.

It was mentioned in an earlier chapter that sleep occurs because of less electrical activity in the current generator, or reticular formation, of the brainstem, and that the less activity there is in the brainstem, the deeper the level of unconsciousness, with sleep being a relatively mild level of unconsciousness. Although this is true, it is not entirely true, as sleep is also an active process that results from increased electrical activity in an area of the brainstem that actively inhibits the electrical activity in the current generator and this "forces" sleep to occur. This phenomenon of "forcing" unconsciousness only occurs with sleep and not with other forms of unconsciousness, all of which are due only to decreased electrical activity in the brain and brainstem.

There are five stages of sleep, each of which is necessary in a typical night's sleep in order to feel well-rested and "rejuvenated" the next day. The first four stages of sleep are arbitrarily designated by patterns that appear on an electroencephalogram (EEG). That is, as the wave pattern changes to indicate deeper and deeper levels of sleep, the corresponding stages of sleep are assigned. Stage 1 of sleep refers to a fairly light sleep while stage 4 of sleep refers to a very deep sleep. REM sleep (rapid eye movement sleep) resembles the awake state on the EEG tracing, and is called "active" sleep because of this.

In order for the brain to be completely de-toxified from the effects of being awake for 16 or more hours during the day, the brain must go through all four of the passive stages of sleep from light sleep to deep sleep. It has been shown that if people are prevented from having REM sleep, they suffer no physiologic or psychologic effects. However, once they are allowed to sleep normally, they will spend more time in REM sleep for a few days after being deprived of it. We dream during all five stages of sleep, but can only remember dreams that occur during REM sleep and stages 1 and 2 of passive sleep. Most of the rejuvenation of the brain takes place during the deeper stages of sleep, including stage 3 and stage 4, a point that will become important when discussing some of the causes for daytime sleepiness. Nightmares and sleep walking also occur during stages 3 and 4 of sleep, as does bed-wetting.

REM sleep is "dream" sleep. It is usually easy to tell when someone is in REM sleep because, as the name suggests, the side to side eye movements under their closed eyelids can be easily seen. REM sleep is also called "active" sleep because the dreams that occur during this period of sleep are quite vivid. In fact, it is known that when we go into REM sleep, our brain becomes "disconnected" from our bodies such that we are unable to move anything but our eyes during REM sleep. It is felt that this is a protective mechanism to keep us from injuring ourselves by violent movements in the bed while we are having the active dreams of REM sleep. No one knows why we have REM sleep. As mentioned above, it is not necessary for rejuvenating the brain.

Each night when we go to sleep, we go through the various stages of sleep, starting with stage 1 and progressing through stage 4, which is then followed by REM sleep. This normal pattern is fairly the same in all people during normal sleep. It is repeated over and over throughout the night. Deviation from this pattern can be responsible for sleep abnormalities, including both insomnia and hypersomnia, as will be seen when discussing the various causes of the different sleep abnormalities.

Although all the various stages of sleep are important for feeling well rested the following day, if one does not reach stage 3 or stage 4 of sleep, he or she is the most likely to feel tired the next day.

We will now discuss the various causes and treatments of abnormal sleep, starting with insomnia, which is by far the more common complaint, and then going on to hypersomnia.

INSOMNIA

Although it may sound unbelievable, about 10% of people have chronic insomnia. Insomnia may result from worry, stress, anxiety, depression, medications, pain, sleep apnea, shift work or a change in time zones, age, or side effects of other medical problems.

There are three types of insomnia. These include difficulty falling asleep, difficulty staying asleep (which usually means that a person has no trouble going to sleep but once he or she awakens, it is very difficult to get back to sleep), and frequent awakenings during the night, although the person is usually able to fall back asleep after each awakening. We will see that the various causes of insomnia mentioned above may relate to one or more of these three types of insomnia.

Worry, stress and anxiety all seem to cause a difficulty with falling asleep. These emotional states cause insomnia because all three cause an increase in the electrical activity of the brain. When this excess electrical activity finds its way down to the wires of the reticular activating system of the brainstem where the sleep state is controlled, it keeps the reticular activating system stimulated and sleep can then not begin. One may wonder why worry, stress, and anxiety cause increased electrical activity in the brain. This is because when someone feels one of these emotions, what is really happening in the brain is that certain memories pertaining to the cause of the particular emotion are being continuously activated by electric current that originates in the emotional area of the brain by a conscious effort on the part of the person who is worried or anxious about something. For example, if a person has a presentation to make the next day, he or she might continue to think about the presentation after going to bed if it is felt that either the person is not well prepared for the presentation or if there is an anxiety associated with the possibility of making a mistake when giving the presentation in front of a large group of people. In the brain, this anxiety is manifested as increased electrical activity originating in the emotional center of the brain, which then continues to send electrical impulses from the wires in this area to the memory branches that pertain to memories associated with the presentation. The ideal result should be that the person rehearses over and over what will be presented the next day until he or she is satisfied, and then falls asleep. Unfortunately, with all of this electrical activity being generated in the emotional area of the brain, some of it is bound to travel to other areas of the brain and brainstem and ultimately ends up in the reticular activating system where it keeps the person from falling asleep.

Depression can also cause difficulty with falling asleep if the depression is caused from external causes, such as the death of a loved one, losing a job, or getting a divorce. If depression is caused from internal problems, such as a chemical imbalance within the brain, this usually results in a difficulty with staying asleep.

The first type of depression, which results from external origins, causes insomnia for the same reasons as stress or anxiety explained above. That is, the person's emotional center in the brain stays continually activated electrically to send impulses to the memory areas pertaining to the memories of the depressing situation and some of this electrical activity finds its way to the reticular activating system of the brainstem where it prevents sleep from occurring.

Internal depression causes difficulty staying asleep because the chemical imbalance that triggers an internal depression can cause the wires of the brain to be more easily stimulated with less electrical current, the result of which is more electrical activity in the brain with any given stimulus. Therefore, with this increased electrical activity in the brain from even a small stimulus, such as turning over in bed at night while asleep (which causes the mechanoreceptors in the skin to send sensory impulses to the brainstem which normally fizzle out when a person is asleep, but don't when a person has a chemical imbalance that lets these sensory impulses travel all the way to the cortex of the brain where they are normally interpreted), the person is bound to wake up and then is unable to fall back asleep until all of the electrical activity eventually dies down. Sometimes this can take a very long time, especially if the emotional areas of the brain become activated when the person wakes up and then worries about not being able to fall back asleep, for the reasons stated earlier.

The treatment for all of the above causes of insomnia, including stress, anxiety, internal depression, and external depression is anti-depressant medications, none of which are addictive. There are about 30 or 40 different ones on the market and in order to find which one works the best, one has to try them and see. (I have found that amytriptyline and trazadone seem to work the best for my patients. They are taken about 20 to 30 minutes before going to bed.) All of the medications that are specifically made to help a person fall asleep and are referred to as "sleeping pills" are addictive and have no place in the treatment of chronic insomnia as they will only ease the problem for a few days or weeks until the person gets used to them. At this point, either the dosage has to be increased or the person has to stop using them, which causes a rebound insomnia that is worse. This second problem of addiction with these medications can be very difficult to deal with, in my experience.

Medications can cause insomnia. Some of the various heart medications and high blood pressure medications are notorious for this, but these are by no means the only ones. It is not too difficult to determine whether a medication is the cause of insomnia because there is usually a cause and effect relationship between the starting of a medication and a resulting insomnia. Usually other medications can be substituted for the offending ones.

Medications cause insomnia in much the same way as a chemical imbalance. That is, because of their effects on the chemicals that allow the current to spread from one wire to the next within the brain, the wires are more easily stimulated. This interrupts the normal dissipation of sensory electrical current that arrives at the brainstem while asleep and allows it to spread to other areas of the brain. This excess electrical activity in the brain either awakens the person more easily from sleep or prevents him or her from going to sleep.

Pain causes a frequent awakening type of insomnia. People who have arthritis, ulcers, angina, prostate problems that require frequent trips to the bathroom at night, or other chronic pain syndromes may complain of insomnia.

Pain wires are very "persistent" in getting their sensory messages delivered to the brain so that the brain can do something to correct the problem that is triggering the pain. This is a protective mechanism and helps with self-preservation, since the whole purpose of the sensation of pain is to let us know that something is wrong somewhere in our bodies. When pain impulses traveling up the sensory wires reach the sleep centers of the brainstem, they override the impulses whose current generation causes the sleep state, and the person immediately awakens.

The treatment for this cause of insomnia is to eliminate the cause of the pain, and if this is not possible, then to inhibit the current from reaching the brain that travels up the pain wires. Narcotic pain relievers do just that. Unfortunately, the body adapts to these medications so that more and more of them are required for the relief of the pain to the point where they may simply stop working altogether. Then, if they are discontinued, the person suffering from the pain has even more pain because of the way the body adapts to these medications by increasing the number of pain wire endings in the brain to counteract the decreased number of pain signals reaching the brain when the narcotics are first taken. (Remember that the brain is very adaptable to various situations and can add more branches to the wires as needed. It cannot, however, add to the total number of wires.) Sometimes, changing back and forth from one pain reliever to another every few weeks can circumvent this problem if the two pain relievers cause slightly different types of responses in the brain. That is, when the brain counteracts the pain-reducing qualities of one pain reliever after a few weeks, the other can be substituted for awhile so that the changes in the brain from the first medication can resolve, since, once the cause for the changes in the number of branches on the wires is eliminated, the excess branches are slowly eliminated also.

Sleep apnea is a fairly unique cause of insomnia in that it prevents a person from reaching the deeper stages of sleep, including both stage 3 and stage 4 of sleep. Because of this, the person does not feel well-rested when he or she awakens in the morning. "Apnea" refers to the cessation of breathing that occurs in some people when they reach the deeper stages of sleep, which then causes them to awaken enough to start breathing again. They cannot get beyond stage 2 of sleep before this phenomenon occurs, and since most of the rejuvenation process of sleeping occurs during stages 3 and 4 of sleep, they never feel well-rested.

Sleep apnea can occur for two reasons. The first, which is called obstructive sleep apnea, occurs because of a mechanical problem in the throat where, as the person falls into the deeper stages of sleep, the muscles that surround the breathing tubes become more and more relaxed to the point where they obstruct the breathing tubes and no air is allowed to get to the lungs when the person tries to take a breath. This causes the person to momentarily awaken somewhat, causing him or her to revert back to stage 1 or 2 of sleep, and then the whole process starts over again. Almost without exception, people who have obstructive sleep apnea are obese with lots of extra fatty tissue surrounding the neck and breathing apparatus such that when the muscles in this area relax during the deeper stages of sleep, this extra tissue gets in the way of breathing. They are almost always loud snorers too.

The second type of sleep apnea, central sleep apnea, is caused from an abnormality in the breathing center, which is located below the sleep center in the brainstem, and occurs because, as the person falls into the deeper stages of sleep, the automatic control over breathing regulation stops working properly for unknown reasons. Occasionally, when someone has a stroke in this area of the brainstem, central sleep apnea can result.

Of the two types of sleep apnea, obstructive sleep apnea is far more common than central sleep apnea. More than 90% of sleep apnea is of the obstructive type.

It was once thought that sleep apnea was very rare, but it is being found that at least the obstructive type sleep apnea is not all that uncommon. In fact, there are more and more sleep labs springing up all over the country for the purpose of diagnosing sleep apnea. (Of course, these labs are quite lucrative for their owners too, which may also explain the increase in their numbers.)

A polysomnogram is the study that is used to diagnose sleep apnea. It is performed overnight in a sleep lab. The patient has various monitors attached to his or her body to record various parameters. These include chest, abdominal, nose, heart, eye, leg, and scalp monitors. There is also an oxygen sensor that tells if the patient's oxygen level in the body falls dangerously during an apnea episode.

The chest, abdominal, and nose monitors help to tell whether apnea is central or obstructive in origin. That is, if the apnea is obstructive in origin, the chest and abdominal monitors will show that the patient is trying to breathe air into the lungs while asleep. But if the nose monitor shows that no air is passing through the nose or mouth, then this means that even though the lungs are trying to expand in order to bring in air, something is blocking the air from getting to the lungs. Hence, the diagnosis of obstructive sleep apnea is made.

The eye monitor helps to tell when the patient is in REM sleep as this monitor keeps track of eye movements, which are very minimal except when one is in REM sleep.

The leg monitor keeps tabs on how restless a patient is during the sleep state. If this monitor shows an excess of movement of the legs during the sleep state, this is often associated with not reaching the deeper stages of sleep and the person doesn't feel well rested the next day. The cause for this increased leg movement is invariably from stress, anxiety, depression, or chronic pain syndromes.

The scalp monitors record the electrical activity of the brain and show which stages of sleep a person is in at any given time, since each of the five stages of sleep has its own peculiar electrical pattern. The heart monitor is used mainly as an aid for the scalp monitors so that if any suspicious activity is seen in the scalp recording, it can be readily determined if the suspicious activity is only electrical activity from the heart that is being transmitted along the surface of the body to the scalp monitors and is thus, only artifact.

The treatment for both types of sleep apnea is the same. It includes placing a small mask over the nose at night while the patient sleeps that forces air into the lungs. This device will push the air past a blocked airway quite well. It also seems to provide enough oxygen for patients who have a central sleep apnea where the brainstem is not telling them to breathe when they reach stage 3 or 4 of sleep. Although it would seem that just wearing a device such as this would keep someone from falling asleep at all, people actually do quite well with this system and the resulting improvement in their sleep is frequently very dramatic.

Changes in time zones, such as is seen with people who work for the airlines, and changes in shifts can cause insomnia. Our bodies get used to going to sleep at a certain time each night, and when we deviate from this, insomnia can result.

Age can affect our sleep patterns. As we get older, we do not require as much sleep. In my practice, I see several older patients each month who complain of not sleeping long enough. Usually, they will go to bed about 8 or 9PM and wake up about 1 or 2AM. They lie in bed the rest of the night trying to fall back asleep, but can't. Five or six hours of sleep a night is normal for someone over the age of sixty. Unfortunately, older people are usually not as active as younger people and don't seem to have as many goals to reach. This can result in boredom, especially after retirement, that causes viewing sleep as an "escape" from the boredom. Instead of sleeping less, they would prefer to sleep more than when they were younger. This problem can be very difficult to treat since, physiologically, there is really nothing "wrong" with the patient. Although medications can be used to help a person sleep longer, all of the medications that will solve this problem are addictive, meaning that they will only work for a relatively short time before they either have to be increased in their dosages or discontinued. When they are eventually discontinued, the patient will have a rebound insomnia because of the fact that these medications all cause a change in the architecture of the brain to make the brain more able to respond to the decrease in current that results from the medications. Then when the medications are no longer used, all of the adaptations that were made by the brain cause it to be more active than normal until it can re-adapt to how it was before the medications were used. This can take up to several weeks, and during this time, the patient has more of a problem with being able to sleep than he or she had in the first place. In my experience, the best treatment for the decreased need for sleep with age is to try to get the patient to go to bed later at night. If patients go to bed around midnight and then sleep until 6AM, they seem to feel more rested than if they go to bed at 8PM and wake up at 2AM. This may have something to do with waking up at a time when it is starting to get light outside, which may subjectively cause one to feel that he or she slept longer, as opposed to waking up 4 or 5 hours before daybreak and lying in bed until daybreak.

Insomnia may be caused as a side effect of other medical problems. For instance, people who have an overactive thyroid are prone to insomnia. The treatment for this, of course, is to treat the underlying condition.

HYPERSOMNIA

Hypersomnia is not nearly as prevalent as insomnia. I would estimate that for every person that I see with a complaint of hypersomnia, I see 60 to 70 patients with a complaint of insomnia.

The causes for hypersomnia can include some of the same, generally, as for insomnia. These would include such things as medications, sleep apnea, and the side effects of other medical conditions. Narcolepsy is probably the most well known of the causes for hypersomnia, even though it is rare. Other sleep disorders due to excessive sleep from unknown causes in the brain are called pathologic sleep disorders.

Narcolepsy is very rare, but it is an interesting sleep disorder because of the symptoms associated with it. There are four main characteristics associated with narcolepsy. These are cataplexy, which is a phenomenon that causes a person to lose consciousness, especially when he or she begins laughing, but can also occur with other emotional changes, daytime somnolence, which indicates that a person may fall asleep very easily during the day, even if a good night's sleep was obtained the previous night, REM onset sleep, both at night and during the day, if one takes naps during the day because of this disease (normally, REM sleep does not occur until a person has been asleep for about 90 minutes), and finally, sleep paralysis, which occurs because of the sleep onset REM activity. (Remember, when a person is in REM sleep, the brain is effectively "disconnected" from the body so that as the person dreams, he or she is unable to move around in the bed and injure himself or herself if an attempt is made to act out the active dreams that occur in the REM stage of sleep.)

Narcolepsy has been shown to be genetic in origin. At one time it was thought to also arise from head injuries, especially when the brainstem is injured, since it is in the brainstem that the abnormality that causes narcolepsy is located. However, it has never been able to be shown that narcolepsy can arise from head injuries. The treatment for narcolepsy includes daily amphetamines, such as methylphenidate. This only works part of the time, however, and in fact, this disease is not very easy to treat successfully. The episodes of cataplexy can be treated with imipramine, an anti-depressant. This medication, unlike the medications used for the narcolepsy, do work relatively well to stop the cataplectic episodes.

Just as medications can cause insomnia, they can also cause hypersomnia. Medications that slow down a person's metabolism have a tendency to cause sleepiness. Seizure medications are notorious for causing sleepiness because of the general way in which they work to decrease the electrical activity of the brain to prevent seizures. Unfortunately, this decrease in electrical activity in the cortex of the brain where seizures originate also decreases the electrical activity in the brainstem where sleep is controlled, which results in hypersomnia. Some blood pressure medications have a tendency to make a person sleepy also.

Some medical conditions can cause excess sleepiness. Just as an overactive thyroid can cause insomnia, an underactive thyroid can cause hypersomnia. People with kidney disease may become excessively sleepy when the toxic products that are usually filtered out by the kidneys are allowed to circulate through the body. Hypersomnia that results from medical conditions is usually not too difficult to diagnose with simple, routine blood tests. The treatment for these causes of hypersomnia is to correct the underlying medical problem, if possible.

Sleep apnea causes insomnia because it prevents a person from reaching stage 3 and 4 of sleep, as mentioned earlier, but it also causes excessive daytime sleepiness because the person is not getting normal sleep at night. The treatment for this is the forced air mechanism mentioned in the section on insomnia.

Pathologic sleep disorders encompass the remaining causes for excessive daytime somnolence, even when a person gets a good night's sleep the previous night. That is, the person with a pathologic sleep disorder sleeps well at night but also has difficulty staying awake during the day. In effect, this cause of hypersomnia is similar to narcolepsy but does not have the associated sleep onset REM activity.

The pathologic sleep disorders, as well as narcolepsy, are diagnosed with a multiple sleep latency test. This is essentially an EEG that is done for 20 minutes, a total of four times, with a 10 or 15 minute interval in between each 20 minute session where the patient is awakened if he or she has fallen asleep during that session. If the person falls asleep within 5 minutes of starting a session on at least two of the sessions, this is classified as a pathologic sleep disorder. If REM sleep is seen during these sessions when a patient falls asleep within 5 minutes, then he or she is likely to have narcolepsy.

In summation, sleep disorders include both difficulty with obtaining sleep and difficulty with staying awake during the day. Difficulty with obtaining sleep is much more predominant than difficulty with staying awake. Most of the time, stress and medications are the causes for insomnia, while medications alone are the usual causes of hypersomnia.

Chapter 10

Chapter 11
SEX PROBLEMS

From an evolutionary standpoint, the only goal of all species of plants and animals is to perpetuate the species by reproducing. If a species is not able to do this adequately, it will become extinct, no matter how highly developed and advanced its intellectual ability may be. With this in mind, it may be easier to understand that most of our problems with sexual dysfunction are self-caused, either because of psychological difficulties or because of medications, rather than from failure of the reproductive organs themselves. That is, because of the importance of reproduction for survival of our species, the actual mechanism for getting the sperm to the egg and the nurturing of this union for nine months is very well protected with various back-up systems to prevent it from failing.

In order for reproduction to occur, there has to be a driving force to cause a male and a female to want to create offspring. Traditionally, this driving force for women has been thought of as resulting from the hormonal influences of nurturing and caring for a child while, for men, the driving force has been thought to result from the intense pleasure derived during the sex act.

It has been known for a long time that nearly 100% of men masturbate, but surprisingly, through polls and studies done over the last 10 to 15 years, it has been found that 70 to 75% of women also masturbate. With the knowledge that sexual pleasure is also very important to women as well as men, this leads to psychological pressures for both men and women to "perform" well during the sex act. This pressure to perform leads to problems with sexual dysfunction in many cases.

In this chapter, we will discuss the causes for sexual dysfunction. As mentioned above, most of the problems related to sexual dysfunction are derived from medications and psychologic causes. However, certain medical conditions can also lead to sexual dysfunction. First, the mechanisms involved in the performance of the sex act will be described, and then the problems that can result from failure of any part of this system will be discussed.

Although it may appear to be somewhat sexist in that the description of the mechanism involved in the sex act pertains almost exclusively to the male, this is necessary because of the sequence of events that must actively take place in the male reproductive organs for the act to occur. (The active role played by the female reproductive organs occurs mainly after an egg has been fertilized.)

The autonomic nervous system is involved in the events pertaining to the sex act. As you may recall from a previous chapter, the autonomic nervous system is involved in "automatic" type behavior that we don't have to voluntarily control, such as regulating our heart rate, moving food through our intestines, dilating our pupils in darkness and constricting them in intense light, and other bodily functions.

There are two areas of the nervous system that are involved in initiating the sex act. One is in the brain and the other is in the lowest section of the spinal cord.

The sex area of the brain is located in the deeper areas of the brain below the cortex, and is stimulated by erotic thoughts that originate in the sensory cortex of the brain in response to various stimuli, such as erotic pictures or simply thinking erotic thoughts. These erotic thoughts are actually electric currents that are directed from the memory branches that pertain to erotica to the deeper areas of the brain that then begin the preparation of the penis for the sex act. In this deeper area of the brain, electrical impulses are initiated that travel down the spinal cord, then out to the wires around the blood vessels in the penis where they cause contraction of the muscles in the blood vessels of this area. This results in an inability of the blood to drain out of the penis, even though blood continues to be pumped into it from the heart, which causes the penis to harden in the same way that a bicycle tire hardens when air is pumped into it. This whole process, of course, is necessary to enable penetration into the vagina.

The process of hardening of the penis can also occur without any initiation from the brain. In these cases, mechanical stimulation of the penis sends electrical impulses from the wires in the mechanoreceptors in the penis to the spinal cord at its lowest levels, which then connect directly to wires in this area of the spinal cord that control constriction of the blood vessels of the penis and cause the hardening process to begin as explained above. In men who have spinal cord damage above this level, such that information can not travel from the brain to the penis or from the penis to the brain, this "reflex" type erection from stimulation of the penis can sometimes still allow enough hardening for penetration of the vagina. In this situation where there is a spinal cord lesion that prevents information from being sent from the penis to the brain and from the brain to the penis, the sex act is usually performed for the purpose of procreation rather than recreation because there can be no orgasmic pleasure derived from the sex act.

This is because "pleasure" can only be experienced in the brain, and in this example, the brain is not able to receive the electric signals for pleasure from the sex glands during the sex act. Sperm can still be produced and ejaculation can still occur, however, without the brain's input. (Remember that the main goal of all species is to reproduce to perpetuate the species and this may be one of our "back-up" systems referred to in the beginning of this chapter.)

In a normal reproductive system, the brain always takes precedence over the spinal cord system mentioned above. For instance, even if the penis is stimulated manually such that erection occurs, if a man has pain in another part of the body not even related to the sex system, the brain can become preoccupied with the pain signals reaching it to the point where the sex act cannot go on to completion. In these cases, even though the lower spinal cord could cause ejaculation to occur, the brain overrides this process and prevents erection and ejaculation from continuing. This same problem can occur if the brain is preoccupied by some emotional crisis, such as stress about one's job, depression about a loved one who may be ill, and so on. In all of these cases, the electric current in the brain is diverted away from the sex area in the deeper areas of the brain and redirected to the memory branches of the person's job or the loved one who is ill. At the same time, there is current directed to areas of the brainstem and spinal cord to actively shut down activity that is not directly related to the present emotional "crisis", hence the inability to complete the sex act to orgasm.

We will now discuss problems that are related to the mechanics of the sex act and then we will discuss problems that relate to inability to reach orgasm.

The mechanics of the sex act pertains to the ability of the penis to penetrate the vagina. As mentioned above, problems with this part of the sex act usually mean an inability to have an erection. In some cases, however, penetration can be prevented by a lack of lubrication from within the vagina, or from vaginal spasms.

Artificial lubricants usually work quite well to overcome the problems of a "dry" vagina. Vaginal spasms may be more difficult to treat. Usually, carbamazepine or clonazepam can be used to correct this problem. Both of these medications work by inhibiting abnormal, self-generated electric currents from traveling down the peripheral wires to the muscles. These medications seem to inhibit only these self-generated impulses while leaving the normal impulses triggered by the brain to move muscles intact.

The most common cause of inability to develop or maintain an erection is medications. In fact, when a patient complains of inability to have an erection, the first question I ask him is what medications he is currently taking. Blood pressure medications are probably the most notorious for causing an inability to have an erection. This is most unfortunate as many men will discontinue these medications for this very reason which then predisposes them to having strokes from the high blood pressure that results. (If a blood pressure medication is discontinued suddenly without tapering it off, a rebound high blood pressure that is higher than would normally exist without the blood pressure medications will result for a period of time, and this is when a stroke is most likely to occur.)

Anti-depressants can also cause inability to have an erection. This is because they affect the electric current in the brain by altering the concentration of the chemicals that control the spreading of the current from the end of one wire to the beginning of the next wire and may interrupt current traveling to the sex center of the brain in this way.

Inability to have an erection can result from other medical conditions that affect the normal circulation of the blood. These would include diabetes, heart disease, and high blood pressure. Diabetes and high blood pressure affect the ability of the blood vessels to respond to the current that travels down the peripheral wires to the muscles that surround the blood vessels such that when the sex area of the brain sends the message to constrict the blood vessels in order for the penis to harden from the inability of the blood to escape from it, the blood vessels cannot respond to this message and an erection does not occur. Heart disease causes inability to have an erection because of the heart's inability to keep forcing blood into the penis as it begins to harden. This is because of the back pressure that results. That is, the heart is too weak to overcome the back pressure from the hardening penis and this prevents it from getting hard enough to penetrate the vagina. The treatment for inability to have an erection because of these chronic medical conditions is to treat the underlying medical condition, if this is possible.

When a patient complains of inability to have an erection, after it is determined that it is not because of a medication he is taking and it is not from one of the chronic medical conditions mentioned above that are notorious for causing inability to have an erection, the next question that is asked concerns whether the patient has early morning erections when he first wakes up, or if he ever has erections that are not precipitated by erotic thoughts. If the answer is that there are never any erections, then a search is made for malfunctions in the sex area of the brain and in the lowest part of the spinal cord. An MRI of the brain or lumbar spinal cord can be done, depending on whether abnormalities on the neurological exam indicate a problem localized to the brain or spinal cord are found. If no abnormalities are found on the neurological exam, then an MRI of both areas may be done to attempt to find the source of the problem. It is important to point out that a mechanical cause for inability to have an erection that is not due to medications being taken, or to one of the medical conditions mentioned above, is so rare that it almost never occurs.

If a patient says that he does have early morning erections on awakening, and erections not associated with erotic thoughts, then there is no "mechanical" cause for the inability to have an erection during the sex act, but rather, a psychological cause. The reasons for this are the same reasons for inability to have an orgasm and affect women as well as men.

Failure to reach orgasm in an otherwise intact sexual system is almost always due to an emotional cause. This can be in the form of stress, worry, or anxiety that may be obvious to the person with this problem, or may be less obvious. In the less obvious cases, a psychiatrist can usually be of assistance in identifying the problem so that it can then be corrected. For instance, if a person has contempt for his or her sex partner for reasons unrelated to sexual matters, it may be difficult for that person to reach orgasm during the sex act with that partner. This is because the emotional areas of the brain send stronger electrical signals to the sex area of the brain that override the incoming electric current from the sex organs. That is, there is electrical current being directed to the sex area of the brain from two different areas, one from the sex organs trying to cause orgasm to eventually occur, and the other from the emotional area of the brain effectively inhibiting any response of the sex area of the brain to sexual stimulation by "tying up" all the available circuits in the sex area. Of course, the current produced in the emotional centers of the brain is not actually "directed" towards the sex area of the brain to stop any sexually related impulses; it is excess electrical activity generated from the emotional area of the brain to all parts of the brain at the same time, and effectively interrupts any incoming sensory signals, which in this case, happens to be sensory signals from the sex organs. If the person were trying to concentrate on some particular piece of information, for instance, at that particular time, rather than trying to perform the sex act, he or she would likely have difficulty concentrating, for the same reason. That is, when trying to direct electric current to the memory branch for the particular piece of information the person is attempting to recall, the current would be interrupted by the current being generated from the emotional area of the brain. (This, as stated in a previous chapter, is what occurs when a person has memory problems when he or she is depressed, worried, or anxious.)

Other emotional states besides contempt for one's sexual partner can cause inability to reach orgasm. Stress, worry, or anxiety from hundreds of other causes can also interrupt orgasm.

Although not as common now as a generation or two ago, inhibition because of sexual taboos can also prevent reaching orgasm by the same mechanism as explained above. That is, the emotional state of "guilt" about sex causes an overriding of the sensory signals from the sex organs and prevents reaching orgasm. It used to frequently be taught by mothers to their daughters that sex was something to be endured rather than enjoyed, and that only "loose" women actually got any enjoyment out of the sex act. As stated in the beginning of this chapter, this attitude is changing.

Primary inorgasmia is an inability to reach orgasm, usually because a person has never had one or only rarely has one. At one time this was thought to be an uncommon occurrence, but has been found to be more prevalent, especially in women. The sex area of the brain apparently has a need to form a "memory" branch for the intense sexual pleasure derived from orgasm, and until this memory branch is created, orgasm cannot be experienced. If this memory branch is not used very often by sending electric current through it occasionally, it may become more difficult to "find" the circuit leading to it. In some people, this memory branch is apparently more difficult to create than in others. However, through more intense, prolonged stimulation or vibration of the clitoris or penis, a first orgasm can essentially always be reached. Successive orgasms then become much easier to attain if stimulation occurs more frequently.

In summation, sexual problems that result from inability to have an erection are almost all due to medications or a chronic medical condition such as diabetes, high blood pressure, or heart disease. Inability to reach orgasm when no mechanical problems occur is almost always due to the emotional area of the brain "overriding" the sexual area of the brain because of stress, worry, anxiety, or inhibition from sexual taboos.

Chapter 11

Chapter 12
PUTTING IT ALL TOGETHER

In the previous chapters, we have seen that everything related to a malfunction in the nervous system has to do with inability of an electrical message to be transmitted from one place to another by way of the living wires that make up the nervous system. An EEG can actually record "shorts" in the wiring of the brain. An MRI or CAT scan can actually show areas where the wires have been destroyed.

It is often difficult for people to accept the fact that the nervous system, especially the brain, does not have some "magical" property that makes it work. In the chapter on headaches, we saw that the pain associated with a headache comes from the brain's interpretation of electrical signals coming from sensory areas around the head. We saw that confusion results from sensory signals arriving at the brain being misdirected or mishandled by the wires that process the incoming signals. In the chapter on memory problems, it was seen that failure to remember events is due to inability to get an electrical impulse to travel up a particular memory branch of one of the memory wires.

Dizziness was seen to occur because of either conflicting electrical signals from the inner ears causing the brain to be unable to process the information accurately, or because of a decreased flow of blood to the brain that prevents the wires from getting enough nutrients to work properly. In the chapter on blackouts, we saw that if there was not enough electrical activity being processed in the brain, or, in the case of seizures, if there is too much electrical activity in the brain, we are rendered unaware of our surroundings. We saw that numbness and tingling were caused from defects in the wires involved in carrying information about the sensation of "touch". Weakness was seen to occur from inability to get an electrical signal to travel all the way from the brain to the muscles without interruption because of an electrical problem somewhere between the brain and the muscles (except in the rare cases where the problem is due to a malfunction in the muscle itself). Tremors were seen to occur because of inability of the wires in the brainstem and cerebellum to properly process the outgoing electrical signals. Pain in the neck and back were seen to occur because of compression of the wires that carry pain impulses to the brain. In the chapter on sleep problems, it was seen that difficulty sleeping is from either excess electrical activity in the brain or because of the effect of medications on the ability of the wires in the brain to function as they were intended. Sex problems were also seen to result from the effects of medications on the wires of the brain that deal with sex. It was also shown that sex problems can result from too much electrical activity in other parts of the brain that interfere with the proper processing of electrical signals related to the sex act. From all of this, it should be seen that everything we feel, think, and do is the result of an electrical signal that passes up or down a living wire in our nervous systems. When we are happy and we laugh, when we are sad and we cry, when we are in love and cannot stop thinking about the person who is the object of this affection, when some of us become murderers and serial killers while others spend their entire lives working to care for less fortunate people in third world countries, it is ultimately because of the way that an electrical signal is handled when it arrives in a particular location in the brain. There is nothing "magical" about this. Because of the way the brain is laid out genetically, along with environmental influences (which are really just sensory signals arriving at the brain for processing over a period of time), we act and react the way we do. If an incoming sensory electrical signal from our eyes for something we have just seen arrives at the emotional center for processing, and it happens to make contact with one specific wire in the emotional area of the brain, it may cause an intense desire to kill someone; whereas, if it makes contact with a neighboring wire in the same area, it may cause us to feel an intense love for the same person.

The brain is the most powerful "piece of equipment" in existence. The most sophisticated computer systems in the world pale in comparison, as they can only manipulate and rearrange data that is fed into them. They are incapable of coming up with new ideas or concepts because they are not "plastic", or capable of change like the brain is. That is, the brain builds new memory branches in response to incoming electrical signals continuously. As these memory branches are made, they may then make contact with other memory branches in close proximity to them such that when an electrical signal travels up one memory branch, it may also stimulate the neighboring memory branch. The stimulation of both of these memory branches at the same time may produce a brand new memory sensation that doesn't have the exact properties of either memory branch as individual branches. The result may be a new idea or concept that has never before occurred in any way to anyone. Computers are not able to do this because they are not "plastic". If a current goes to one area of a computer, it will never vary from the response that it invokes each time it travels down that particular pathway because the pathway is incapable of change. The only way a computer might come up with a new concept would be if someone spills a coke in it and it shorts out just enough that two or more wires are stimulated with electric current at the same time.

It is the way that the wiring of the brain is arranged that makes one a quick or a slow responder to various sensory input. A person who is good at memorizing information can usually recite it back fairly quickly but is less likely to understand what is being recited, while a person who tries to "make sense" of new information is not as likely to be able to repeat it as quickly but will most likely understand it more completely. This is because the person who memorizes something quickly sets up a more direct route from the incoming electrical signal to the memory branch for that information without any deviation to other memory branches that help relate to understanding the information. This more direct route makes the material easier to recall from the memory branch. The person who tries to understand what is being memorized uses more memory branches such that the information can be integrated for association with other learned items in memory, but then this requires a more diffuse pathway to bring this memory back to consciousness. Because of the fact that this person has integrated the information with other memory branches, he or she is better able to explain to someone else what the memorized information means than someone who has only memorized the information for purposes of recital.

The best athletes are those that can react to a situation without having to think about what they are going to do. This is also referred to as "having quick reflexes", which really means that when sensory information is presented to the brain, it makes only a few connections with the wires in the brain before the brain reacts by sending a signal down a movement wire to a muscle. A good example of this is a baseball batter. The sensory information that reaches the brain from the batter's eyes telling him where a ball is being pitched, as well as how fast it is coming, must be processed very quickly in order for him to swing the bat in time to hit the ball. When the coach says to "concentrate", what he is really asking the player to do is to stop all extraneous electrical current in the brain that might divert the incoming sensory information about the pitched ball to other areas of the brain besides to the appropriate movement area.

If all of the above is actually true (and it probably is) then it would be difficult to say that we make "mistakes" because we are "only human". When information of a sensory nature arrives at the brain for processing, it is always processed in an appropriate manner for the way in which the wiring of the brain has been laid out for that particular person. When someone is absent-minded or is unable to remember some piece of information that was expected to be remembered, it is not necessarily a "mistake", but rather that the information was not as important to the person as information that may have been in process in the brain at the same time. In other words, it's not that we make mistakes but rather that at any particular time, we may be processing electrical information that we either consciously or subconsciously feel is more important at that time than the incoming electrical information. At other times, we may make mistakes because we don't possess all the information in our memory branches to make an "informed" decision at that particular time. Still other causes of mistakes may be from conflicting sensory information, such as when the eyes don't focus on something properly. In all these cases, however, the brain is not making any mistakes. It is simply acting in accordance with its architectural makeup upon the sensory information with which it has been provided for processing. Of course, if one uses the definition of "mistake" to mean "any outcome that is not intended", then these are actual mistakes, but the point being made here is that everything that goes on in the brain is for a purpose and is not whimsical.

Although it has been mentioned several times throughout this book, I will mention one last time that the most important message to be conveyed about the way the nervous system and all malfunctions associated with it work is due to the ways in which electrical impulses that are conducted from one wire to the next are handled by the brain, the spinal cord, and the peripheral nerves.

Index

ORDER FORM

TOLL FREE
1-(800) 909-2794
(Have VISA or Mastercard ready)

FAX 1-(912) 261-0085
(include name, address, phone,
VISA or MC number, and expiration date)

POSTAL ORDERS

$14.95
$2.50 shipping
$17.45 total
(Georgia residents add $.75 tax)

SEND TO:

Boxweed Publishing
91 Gould Street
St. Simons Island, GA 31522

UNCONDITIONAL GUARANTEE
If you are not satisfied with this book for any reason,
you may return it at any time for a full refund,
excluding shipping charges. (Book must not be torn,
scuffed, or defaced, however.)